PENGUIN BOOKS

THINK BEFORE YOU SWALLOW

Noel O'Hare is a journalist and columnist who has been writing about health issues for over 20 years. His work has been recognised with numerous awards including the Qantas Media Awards Senior Feature Writer of the Year and the Rosalyn Carter Mental Health Journalism Fellowship. He is best known for his writing in the *New Zealand Listener*, but has contributed to many publications including the UK *Guardian*.

THINK BEFORE YOU SWALLOW

The Art of Staying Healthy in a Health-Obsessed World

Noel O'Hare

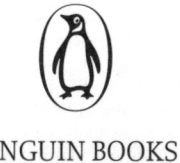

PENGUIN BOOKS

PENGUIN BOOKS
Published by the Penguin Group
Penguin Group (NZ), 67 Apollo Drive, Rosedale,
North Shore 0632, New Zealand (a division of Pearson New Zealand Ltd)
Penguin Group (USA) Inc., 375 Hudson Street,
New York, New York 10014, USA
Penguin Group (Canada), 90 Eglinton Avenue East, Suite 700, Toronto,
Ontario, M4P 2Y3, Canada (a division of Pearson Penguin Canada Inc.)
Penguin Books Ltd, 80 Strand, London, WC2R 0RL, England
Penguin Ireland, 25 St Stephen's Green,
Dublin 2, Ireland (a division of Penguin Books Ltd)
Penguin Group (Australia), 250 Camberwell Road, Camberwell,
Victoria 3124, Australia (a division of Pearson Australia Group Pty Ltd)
Penguin Books India Pvt Ltd, 11, Community Centre,
Panchsheel Park, New Delhi – 110 017, India
Penguin Books (South Africa) (Pty) Ltd, 24 Sturdee Avenue,
Rosebank, Johannesburg 2196, South Africa

Penguin Books Ltd, Registered Offices: 80 Strand, London, WC2R 0RL, England

First published by Penguin Group (NZ), 2007
1 3 5 7 9 10 8 6 4 2

Copyright © Noel O'Hare, 2007

Some of the material in this book appeared in a different form in the
New Zealand Listener.

Designed by Mary Egan
Typeset by Egan Reid Ltd
Prepress by Image Centre
Printed in Australia by McPherson's Printing Group

ISBN: 978-014-300602-2

A catalogue record for this book is available
from the National Library of New Zealand.

www.penguin.co.nz

CONTENTS

Foreword

A journalist once asked footballer George Best if there was any therapy he might still try to kick the booze. His reply was resounding:

> I never wanted to stop. I've had enough of all those patronising so-and-sos trying to tell me I'd have a better life without it. I don't want to live without it. I'm no good without it.

Health professionals tend to feel aggrieved when people like George Best tell them they're patronising. Many feel they have failed in their duty if they do not speak out when they see others 'getting life wrong'. It's easy to understand their hurt and bemusement, but it's a lot harder to understand why health professionals can't work out why rebels like George find them so patronising.

Were they to read *Think Before You Swallow*, they'd get it in a flash.

Today's health systems use technologies that were science fiction 20 years ago – cutting-edge pharmaceuticals, ultra-sophisticated imaging, even face transplants – yet philosophically they're stuck in the dark ages. Despite doing so many other things so well, our health systems never bother to examine their apparently basic beliefs: (1) that health is an objective state; (2) that being healthy means not being diseased, ill or injured; (3) that every rational person must desire health; and (4) that if a person acts in an unhealthy manner it's a health professional's duty to persuade – and if necessary coerce – her into healthy ways.

The problem with these 'official assumptions' is that if health really is an objective state which every rational person must desire, that makes most of us irrational most of the time. If health is a scientific reality then the 'obese' gourmet who lives to eat well must be blind to it; the injury-prone All Black who plays on regardless must be deluded; the drinker who would rather get a daily buzz than live a longer life must be mentally ill; and the 33 per cent of cancer sufferers who cause their own disease are nothing less than wildly irresponsible.

But as everyone outside establishment health systems instinctively knows, not only does a good life involve much more than not being diseased, ill or injured – it almost always requires it.

This sounds illogical to health system 'patronising so-and-sos' because they confuse medical fact with a prescription for living. Medical research shows with increasing precision that there is x per cent chance that y (drinking alcohol, smoking cigarettes, exposure to sunlight) will cause z (liver disease, lung disease, melanoma) – but in life context it doesn't matter how many physical facts are discovered because science has no more authority to tell people how to live than my budgerigar.

The medical view of health is but one philosophy of life amongst a multitude of others – its priorities may be ideal for the conservatively inclined, but are odious or ridiculous to those who aren't.

O'Hare's entertaining and often inspiring folk wisdom simply reminds us of the plain truth that how we live our own lives is up to us.

I can't say that George Best's lifestyle was the wrong choice. How can anyone reasonably be the judge of that? Ultimately, none of us have a clue what the point of living is – though I'm sure it's safe to say (with Noel O'Hare) – that if there is a point it certainly isn't to pursue a medically healthy life above all else.

George Best didn't try to convert anyone else to his philosophy of life, whereas health system 'patronising so-and-sos' want to force us to adopt theirs. But why should we swallow what they want us to? It is infinitely better – whatever sort of life we choose – that we decide how to live for ourselves.

And deciding for ourselves means being able to reach unpressured, informed judgements about the choices that are open to us. Which is precisely what *Think Before You Swallow* offers us.

In more than one sense, George Best swallowed what he wanted and rejected what he didn't. Clearly some of Noel's advice was not for George, but then no advice is right for everyone. However, I strongly suspect he would have liked the book's free-spirited style. I reckon he might even have drunk to it.

Professor David Seedhouse
Director, National Centre for Health and Social Ethics

Introduction

What are you worried about? Cancer? Heart disease? Stroke? Alzheimer's? Apart from diet and exercise, there's not a lot that can be done to reduce your risk of most diseases. However, there is one big health risk that *you* can do something about: naivety. You won't find naivety listed in any medical textbook, but it can have as devastating an effect on your health and well-being as any disease.

> *A man dies after swallowing 10,000 times the daily dose of the antioxidant selenium, recommended as an alternative prostate cancer treatment on the Internet.*

> *A woman with arthritis sees a TV ad for the painkiller Vioxx and asks her doctor if it is right for her. Three years later, she suffers a fatal heart attack.*

> *A parent decides against chemotherapy for her child after a friend tells how her cancer was cured by a homeopath.*

Naivety can be deadly. In the case of the man who swallowed the selenium, he may have assumed that a natural supplement could not cause harm. The woman who took the Vioxx obviously thought that a drug prescribed by her doctor would be safe to use as directed. The parent who put her child's life in jeopardy may have believed that health authorities would not allow alternative healers to practise unless they provided valid treatment.

The irony is that while the Internet allows us easy access to good information on every disease and condition that flesh is heir to, it's never been harder to decide on health care. Two hours on Google may throw up a new approach to treating a disease that your doctor has never heard of, but it would be naive to believe your prowess at Internet searching equates to years of medical training. In the British *Independent* newspaper a doctor wrote about the modern 'heart-sink' patients, the Internet savvy who turn up with a sheaf of printouts: 'Quite recently, one of my own patients took me by surprise by quoting a relevant medical fact, and I found myself asking whether he had a medical degree. "No," he told me, without cracking a smile, "I've got broadband." What usually follows is a burst of disarming intelligence followed by a seamless lapse into gibberish.'

A little knowledge can be a dangerous thing, but that's not to say we shouldn't try to be better informed. It would also be naive to wish for a return to the days when you could place all your faith in your doctor, who mumbled some impenetrable medical jargon and, as humorist Dave Barry put it, 'wrote out a prescription in a Secret Medical Code that neither you nor the CIA could understand. The only person who could understand it was Mr DiGiacinto, who ran the Armonk Pharmacy . . .'

Health care is no longer so straightforward, if indeed it ever was. Medicine and marketing are now so closely intertwined that it's hard to tell one from the other. With their vast resources and influence, the pharmaceutical industry plays a major role in setting the health agenda. Many medical experts who make the decisions in bodies such as the World Health Organisation and the US National Institutes of Health now take money from drug companies. Drug marketing influences every aspect of health from the clinical testing of drugs to the medicalisation of common experiences such as unhappiness, shyness and grief. The boundary between illness and what used to be called life is becoming increasingly blurred. In the UK, for example, men are now being treated for postnatal depression.

We are constantly bombarded with information about health. Every week, it seems, the media report a new health scare, a new medical breakthrough, a new sure-fire diet or a newly revised guideline for healthy living. There are more drugs, more treatments, more research than even doctors find it possible to keep up with. Health has also become a minefield of competing claims, contradictory opinions, and marketing masquerading as health advice. It poses dangers for the naive and ill-informed. Without a context in which to judge claims and information, they put their health at risk.

My aim in writing this book is to help people make better decisions about their health care. There is no formula that will cover all situations, but it's possible to apply some basic principles when reaching a decision. For example, when deciding whether or not to take a particular medication, it's useful to bear in mind that new is not always better though that's usually true with most consumer products. Public Citizen, the independent US watchdog group, recommends waiting seven years before taking a newly approved drug unless it's a breakthrough drug or has documented advantages over older, proven drugs. It's usually during the first seven years that problems show up and drugs are taken off the market because they have been proven dangerous to patients. In 1999, rofecoxib was approved as safe and effective by the US Food and Drug Administration (FDA) and, marketed as Vioxx, quickly became a worldwide top-seller. In 2004 it was withdrawn from the market after many reports of cardiovascular side effects; an estimated 140,000 heart attacks and 56,000 deaths have since been attributed to its use.

As a health writer and columnist for over 20 years, I've learned the value of retaining a healthy scepticism about claims made for both conventional and alternative treatments. I've seen how doctors and other health professionals defend their entrenched positions even when the evidence clearly suggests they are wrong. I know that public relations agencies, acting for drug companies, now have an influential role in deciding which health stories appear in the media because I've been approached many times to write such stories myself. I've interviewed alternative health practitioners and been astounded by their arrogance, complacency, and lack of concern for proof that their treatments work.

This book, however, is not just about conventional and alternative medicine. As Darian Leader and David Corfield remind us in their timely book *Why Do People Get Ill*, the causes of many diseases are often enormously complex interactions between mind and body. The immune system, our defence against illness, is connected to the brain by a complex network of nerves throughout the body. This means 'our mental life could be having a continual effect on our immune system'. Health and well-being depend on more than just taking the right pill or selecting the right therapy. What we do with our bodies and how we manage our thoughts are also important. Family also affects our health and well-being: the genes we carry, our relations with parents and siblings, the people we marry, even our contact with the family pet. Finally, there is the world we live in with all its choices and hazards: the work we do, how we shop for food, the weather, how we travel.

Search for 'personal health' at Amazon.com and you'll be presented with over 20,000 book choices. Yet we've never been healthier. Life expectancy in many industrialised countries has more than doubled over the past century to nearly 80 years and is still rising. People are enjoying better health, with chronic illnesses such as heart disease, lung disease and arthritis affecting us 10 to 25 years later than they used to. The old are less likely to be disabled and more likely to live active pain-free lives. Effective drugs, surgery and medical technology have added immeasurably to the quality of life for many people. Yet, as James Le Fanu has pointed out in his book, *The Rise and Fall of Modern Medicine* 'despite the prodigious medical advances of the post-war years the proportion [of the public] claiming to be "worried" about their health has also risen from 15 per cent to almost 50 per cent over the same period'.

There are many keen to exploit that anxiety: diet gurus, drug companies, supplement sellers, new-age therapists, food manufacturers, advertisers, publishers, insurance sellers, fitness centres, TV producers, editors and more. Though many hazards and risks to health are discussed in this book (ignorance has never been bliss), the aim is to alleviate anxiety not raise it. Most of the time we're better off forgetting about health and instead focusing on living a fulfilling, enjoyable life and connecting with others. Despite the old maxim that if we enjoy it, then it must be bad for us, many of the things that give us real satisfaction in life have proven health benefits. As the studies cited in this book show, taking it easy, hanging out with friends, helping others, enjoying good food and wine, being in a loving and lasting relationship, will do more for our health and well-being than a lifetime of gym exercise, cholesterol monitoring, macrobiotic dieting and the reading of self-actualisation manuals.

Since pleasure and fun are indispensable to health and well-being, I did not want this book to be an exception. So, as well as serious research, there are digressions, asides, anecdotes, trivia, and other miscellanea because writers are entitled to have fun too. Among the things you'll learn, for example, are:

- how to smell six years younger
- how to get bigger tips if you wait on tables
- how to boost your immunity against colds by watching a video
- how to take your hypochondria to the next level.

Think Before You Swallow: The Art of Staying Healthy in a Health-Obsessed World is not a self-help book, though I hope you will find some of the information helpful. There are no habits to acquire or shortcomings to overcome, no quizzes to show how much you need to improve, no lists to memorise or steps to take, no negative thoughts to banish or daily affirmations to make. Well, okay, maybe one. Repeat in the presence of a stranger: *Every day in every way this book just gets better and better.*

Body

I stand in awe of my body.

HENRY DAVID THOREAU
US AUTHOR AND TRANSCENDENTALIST (1817–1862)

ONE

Never Supersize Your Wardrobe

It's a little-studied phenomenon that the longer you leave clothes at the back of the wardrobe, the smaller they get. Over a number of decades, the shrinkage can be incredible. Recently I came across a favourite jacket that I'd last worn in my twenties. It still looked stylish but a 12-year-old would have had difficulty squeezing into it. For the most part, though, clothes that don't fit are a sign you're gaining weight, not a wardrobe malfunction.

Clothes are body sensors alerting us to our increasing bulk. Opting for baggy clothing is like living in a house without smoke alarms. Cutting back on food when our waistbands start to feel tight may be one of the simplest and best ways to stop gaining weight. In his book, *Fatland*, Greg Critser cites an experiment by obesity expert John Garrow. Garrow was studying the post-weight-loss of two groups of patients who had had their jaws wired. For subjects in one group he fitted a wide nylon cord around their waists, tight enough to make a white line in their flesh. The other group had no waistband fitted. The experiment showed 'striking differences between the two groups': one gained 1.8 kg (3.9 lb) a month, while the group with the tight waistband did not gain any significant weight.

And it's the fat gut that is most likely to harm us. Visceral fat surrounds our major organs and could set us up for heart attacks and other health problems. Visceral fat is not inert blubber: it emits important hormones such as leptin that helps us regulate our weight and appetite, and may also combat depression. Fat has always served a useful function as a storehouse of energy – until now. Who needs a big belly when fast food is available 24/7 delivered to your door?

Body mass index (BMI), the most common method to determine if you're overweight or obese, is a simple mathematical formula based on your height and weight. BMI, though, doesn't take into account lean muscle so if you're a gym junkie you may get a false reading. Pint-sized Sylvester Stallone, for example, would be obese on a BMI chart. A BMI between 25–29.5 means you're officially overweight; anything beyond 30 and you're officially obese. But just because you're overweight doesn't mean you're unhealthy. BMI doesn't take into account the fact that you may be very fit and active. In 1996, the US National Center for Health Statistics analysed dozens of studies involving 600,000 subjects. It concluded that for non-smoking men the lowest mortality was found among those with BMI figures between 23 and 29, meaning the majority of the healthiest men in the survey would be considered overweight.

British scientists using an MRI (magnetic resonance imaging) scanner have found that some people who look thin may be carrying dangerous levels of fat around their organs and in their muscles. Alternatively, people who look fat from the outside may be thin on the inside. MRI scans of Sumo wrestlers have shown that they have very little internal fat even though they get through 5000 calories a day.

As it's unlikely your doctor will agree to an MRI scan at your next check-up (unless you want to pay for it), the best way to determine if you're at risk of carrying too much fat is to get out your tape measure. If you're a male with a waist of 101 cm (40 in) or more, or a woman with a 90 cm (35 in) waistline you may be heading for trouble. A bit of prodding helps: visceral fat tends to make a belly feel firm, rather than flabby.

Even if you've always been a relatively small eater, you can start to gain weight as you move into your forties and beyond. As we age, our metabolism slows, burning up fewer calories. We tend to exercise less and lose more muscle. If we keep on eating the same amount we will inevitably gain weight each year. Over a decade this can be quite substantial. Studies suggest that, on average, women between the ages of 35 and 55 gain about 500 g (1.1 lb) a year. That means the average 55-year-old will have put on 10 kg (22 lb) or more since their thirties. No one knows how much fat is dangerous for a particular individual but, to lower the risk of ill health and save money supersizing your wardrobe, you'd be better off eating less. Eating from smaller plates may help. In middle age your dinner plate should shrink like your libido.

The easiest and quickest way to get back into shape is to cut down on bread, rice, pasta and potatoes, in other words an Atkins-type, low-carb diet. The diet was first popularised in 1869 by William Banting, an English coffin-maker, who by the time he came to occupy one of his own caskets was a very healthy weight. At 62, though, he was in bad shape: he weighed 92 kg (202 lb) and was only 165 cm (5.5 ft) tall. 'I could not stoop to tie my shoes, so to speak, nor to attend to the little offices humanity requires without considerable pain and difficulty which only the corpulent can understand.'

He had tried everything to lose weight: exercise, low-calorie starvation diets, Turkish baths and 'gallons of physic and liquor potassae'. Nothing worked. On top of his weight problem, his sight and hearing were failing. Seeking help for the latter he consulted a distinguished ear, nose and throat specialist, Dr William Harvey. Believing his increasing deafness and obesity may be linked, Harvey advised him to give up starchy and sugary foods: bread, milk, sugar, beer and potatoes, but not excluding 'at dinner two or three glasses of good claret, sherry or Madeira'. By the end of that year Banting had lost 23 kg (50 lb) and 33 cm (13 in) off his waist. It cost him little effort. He had lost weight by a 'system of diet that formerly I would have thought dangerously generous ... The great charm and comfort of the system is, that its affects [sic] are palpable within a week of trial, which creates a natural stimulus to persevere for few weeks more, when the fact becomes established beyond question.' Banting became the first diet guru. His *Letter on Corpulence* had sold 58,000 copies by his death in 1878. The diet became so popular that 'banting' entered the language as a synonym for losing weight.

Banting- and Atkins-style diets can be useful in avoiding moving up a clothes size, but shedding lots of weight may not always be healthy. The link between excess weight and ill health is not as clear as some would have us believe. Excess weight is strongly associated with social class and education. The poor and uneducated are more likely to be fat and unhealthy because their diets are bad, they have less access to medical care, and they are more likely to smoke. They are also more vulnerable to social stress, which studies show impairs immunity. Many of the medical conditions simplistically attributed to excess weight may, in fact, be the result of a range of factors.

Certainly, there is not much evidence that losing weight will help you live longer. A study of the effects of voluntary weight loss in 49,000 overweight men by the US Centers for Disease Control and Prevention showed no overall effect on mortality. Cut down on your calories and you may cut down on your immunity. A University of California study tracked a group of overweight women on a 15-week diet. The diet was nutritionally balanced but was only 50 per cent of the usual energy intake. The researchers found that diet compromised the women's immunity in a number of different ways. The most worrying effect was a 25 per cent reduction in natural killer cells, which destroy infected and cancerous cells.

The key to good health seems to be related more to exercise than to weight control. In an American study of 25,389 men from 1974 to 1995, researchers found that fat men who exercised lived just as long as thinner fit men. The study also showed that thin men who were out of shape were nearly three times as likely to die young as fat men who exercised regularly.

Despite the edicts of the food police, it does not seem to matter much what we eat, so long as we include fruit and vegetables in our diet. For example, a leading study published in the *American Journal of Medicine* found that a low-fat diet had no effect on our chances of getting major diseases. The $415 million federal study followed nearly 49,000 women aged 50 to 79 for eight years. Those who were on a low-fat diet had the same rates of breast cancer, colon cancer, heart attacks and strokes as those who ate whatever they pleased.

Eating healthily can also have its dark side. Seldom mentioned is the obnoxious self-congratulation that comes with sticking to a strict food regime. How righteous you feel tucking into vegetables and brown rice for dinner instead of a fried steak and chips. How you look down on degenerates who wash down Big Macs and French fries with Coke. Nor does it escape your attention that when the Lord wanted to feed the five thousand He didn't order in pizzas with extra mozzarella but chose bread, unrefined wholemeal in those days, and fish rich in Omega 3 oils.

Healthy food can take over your life and become an obsession. American doctor Steven Bratman has even coined a term for the condition: orthorexia nervosa (*ortho* from the Greek meaning 'straight'). 'In its essential character, orthorexia bears many similarities to two named eating disorders: anorexia and bulimia,' says Bratman in his book *Health Food Junkies*. 'Whereas the bulimic and anorexic focus on the quantity, the orthorexic fixates on its quality. All three give food a vastly excessive place in the scheme of life.'

Bratman says that orthorexia starts innocently enough as a desire to overcome chronic illness or improve general health. However, the iron self-discipline needed to change the food habits of a lifetime combined with a grim sense of self-righteousness means that few people are able to make the change gracefully. 'Over time, what to eat, how much and the consequences of dietary indiscretion come to occupy a greater and greater proportion of the day.'

Instead of being something to be enjoyed and savoured, food becomes something to worship, says Bratman. In this kind of 'kitchen spirituality', tucking into a tofu burger and organic salad can seem as laudable as spending a day helping the homeless and the destitute. Indulging in 'forbidden food' comes to be seen as a moral lapse, an occasion for self-loathing, followed by repentance and a return to virtue.

In his book *The Power of Pleasure*, psychologist Dale Airens argues that by indulging in the food you like, you tend to eat less while at the same time feeling more sated. 'Time and again, the best diet turns out to be following your palate and indulging yourself. Indulgence also makes it easier to maintain a sensible weight. An enlightened palate that has learned to thrive on the exquisite automatically guides us to the best foods.'

Eat what you like – and let your clothes be the judge of how much.

TWO

Keep Your Nose Clean

In Nikolai Gogol's famous story, 'The Nose', a St Petersburg civil servant wakes up one morning to discover his nose has disappeared, 'to his unbounded astonishment, there was only a flat patch on his face where the nose should have been!' To millions of people with hay fever and other allergies, having your nose vanish overnight would seem a welcome prospect. The misery of a stuffy, itchy or dripping hooter is only compounded by the cost of medication that brings little relief. The expression 'paying through the nose' is said to have its origins in ninth-century Ireland where the Danes slit the nose of anyone unwilling or unable to pay their taxes. But it could equally have originated with drug companies who exploit allergy sufferers' misery by selling their products at a premium. A 2006 survey of US allergy sufferers found that more than half were unhappy with their medication and 47 per cent were taking up to four different medications to relieve symptoms.

It's no wonder that people are returning to the long-neglected practice of nasal cleansing. Research suggests that regular nose cleaning may be the key to fewer sinus problems and can help ward off infections. The nose guards our respiratory system, moistening, filtering and warming the air we breathe. It traps all the contaminants in the air and adjusts the air temperature to match the body temperature. The mucus membrane that lines the nose produces the mucus to capture the dust, pollen and other particles that can irritate the lungs. The cilia or tiny hairs inside the nose help to move the trapped gunk to the front of the nose or to the back of the throat.

Keeping your nose clean has a long history. It has been a popular yoga practice for about 1500 years. Fishermen have been using salt water to clean their nasal passages for generations (well, it was probably something to do when the fish weren't biting). The practice of nasal cleansing became popular in the West about 100 years ago. In 1895, the *British Medical Journal* thundered in an editorial that the nose was 'one of the dirtiest organs in the body' and 'should be washed daily with saline'. A harsh judgement on a sensitive and undervalued organ that has similarities to the penis and the clitoris. But more about the sexual life of the nose later.

Since every surface of our bodies seethes with bacteria, it's no surprise that the nose harbours millions of microbes, most of which are harmless. However, about one in 10 people carry *Staphylococcus aureus* in their nose. Staph, as it's commonly called, can cause skin and bone infections, pneumonia, bloodstream infections and other illnesses, though most of the infections are minor, such as pimples and boils. Another strain, the dreaded superbug, methicillin-resistant *Staphylococcus aureus* (MRSA), is also carried by many healthy people without causing illness. Chemicals in the mucus dissolve many of the bacteria entering the nose, and bacteria is also killed by stomach acid when transported to the back of the throat and swallowed.

Nasal irrigation helps to get the cilia in the nose moving, dilutes and removes mucus, crusts, pollutants and other debris in the nose, and may improve blood and fluid flow between the nasal lining and the blood vessels and body tissues. Like your dog's nose, your nose functions best if it is moist. A dry nose cannot moisten the air we breathe and is likely to collect crusts and sticky mucus, can cause pain and is more prone to nose bleeding. A saline spray (you can make your own with a quarter teaspoon of salt and a quarter teaspoon of baking powder in a cup of water) will help keep your nose from drying out.

Cleaning your nose is a bit trickier. Though there are plenty of high-tech nasal irrigation devices available, many people use a simple teapot-shaped neti pot. Jala neti, an ancient, yoga-cleansing technique is still widely practised in India. Some doctors say that nasal lavage, to use the medical term, is just as important as hand washing and teeth brushing to overall health. Nasal lavage may reduce the number of colds you get or alleviate allergies such as hay fever by rinsing out pollen dust or other allergy-causing particles that get trapped in the nose. It's also cheaper than resorting to over-the-counter drugs, which may have side effects. Other benefits claimed for nasal lavage include fewer headaches, better concentration, improvement in conditions such as asthma and bronchitis, fewer middle-ear infections and decrease in mouth breathing.

One of the benefits of a clean nose is an improved sense of smell. About 60 per cent of our olfactory genes became redundant when we developed trichromatic vision (sensitivity to blue, green and yellow-red), so our sense of smell is infinitely inferior to that of the humble silkworm, which can smell a female two kilometres away. Nevertheless, our noses are a lot more sensitive than we give them credit for. A top-of-the-range human nose can detect up to 10,000 odours. In the 18th century the nose was an important diagnostic tool for doctors. Some illnesses have a definite aroma. German measles smells like freshly plucked feathers; typhoid like freshly baked bread; smallpox like perspiring geese (admittedly not very helpful if you've never been up close and personal with a sweaty goose). The breath of someone in a diabetic coma smells like apples, and, as every whodunnit fan knows, cyanide poisoning leaves a bitter almond smell.

An over-emphasis on personal hygiene has left us insensitive to the smell of others. All mammals, including humans, have specific odours as distinctive as a fingerprint. In 1908, Helen Keller wrote that despite her blindness she could identify individuals by their 'person-odour'. Mothers can recognise their own newborns by odour, even after exposure for a period as short as 10 minutes. Studies also show that fathers, grandmothers and aunts can identify by smell the clothes first worn by the infant. Some scientists believe that there is some genetic basis for family odour. Dogs, for instance, can track down an unfamiliar twin after a quick sniff of his brother or sister.

And consider the human ability to identify MHC. MHC is short for major histocompatibility complex, a segment of DNA that detects disease structures and alerts the immune system to fight them. Studies with mice show that when given a choice they prefer to mate with a partner whose MHC least overlaps their own. This ensures that the offspring will have a wider range of disease resistance than would be the case if the mating had been, say, between brother and sister. Mice are able to detect a prospective mate's MHC by sniffing their urine.

Amazingly, humans can also discriminate between the

urine of mice with different MHC by smell alone. If humans are able to detect small differences in the immune systems of mice, can they also detect MHC in human body odour? Researchers at the University of Bern carried out a study with 100 university students from different campuses. The men were asked to sleep in cotton T-shirts for two nights and refrain from using deodorants or eating spicy foods. The women in the study were then asked to rate the shirts for 'sexiness', 'pleasantness' and 'intensity of smell'. Overall, the women preferred those scents from men whose MHC profiles varied most from their own. (The Swiss researchers also found that women taking oral contraceptives reported reverse preferences.)

Couples who suffer repeated spontaneous abortions tend to share more of their MHC than couples whose pregnancies are carried to full term. The Swiss team speculates that the reason for some infertility problems is that women's bodies unconsciously reject fertilisation because in our evolutionary past offspring with inferior immune systems would not have survived to adulthood.

'All the evidence ... indicates that humans have a highly active scent producing apparatus which seems to be geared to reproductive biology,' says zoologist Michael Stoddart in his book, *The Scented Ape: The Biology and Culture of Human Odour.*

The nose is also affected by sexual arousal. Like the genitals and the nipples, the nasal septum – the part that separates the nostrils – is made of erectile tissue. Honeymoon rhinitis, stuffiness caused by sexual activity, is a well-known condition. Viagra also affects the erectile tissue in the nose, and a nose with a hard-on is not a happy nose. Nasal stuffiness is a common side effect, but Viagra has also been known to cause severe nosebleeds. In many ancient cultures adulterers were punished by having their nose cut off, a penalty that created a market for plastic surgery. The first nose job was done in India about 800 BC.

It may be that we are led by the nose in our choice of sexual partner. Writer George Simenon, the creator of Maigret, who claimed to have slept with 10,000 women, seemed to have had a nose for sex. In *The Man Who Wasn't Maigret*, Simenon's biographer Patrick Marnham speculates that the writer's sexual vigour may have been a consequence of the family's acute sense of smell. 'Was George Simenon fated all his life to be led by the nose? Certainly his earliest descriptions of sexual interest were linked to the sense of smell, notably the market women described in the early teenage novel *Johan Pinaguet*.' It's known that about a quarter of people with smell disorders lose their sex drive.

Wilhelm Fliess, the ear, nose and throat specialist who was a close friend of Sigmund Freud, believed there was a close connection between the nose and the genitals. Fliess's theory never won acceptance, but the idea that the vomeronasal organ, or VNO, in the nose can detect chemical signals passed between humans is gaining ground. The human vomeronasal organ, two tiny receptors that exist about a centimetre inside the nose, were thought, however, to be vestigial.

Scientists assumed that since humans started to walk upright, away from the source of many odours, our sense of smell has long ceased to influence behaviour. However, some courtship customs suggest otherwise. In rural Austria, girls used to keep a slice of apple in their armpits during dances to offer to their swains afterwards. A famous story in the psycho-sexual literature of the 19th century is of a peasant lad who kept a handkerchief there and used it to wipe the sweat from the faces of his dancing partners. Instead of asking 'Prithee, Tom, where doth thy keep thine hankies – in thy bleedin' armpit?', they apparently all said 'Your place or mine?'.

Women have a more acute sense of smell than men. They are particularly sensitive to musky-smelling substances, especially boar taint substance (secreted in the urine of boars), exaltolide (a synthetic musk), and civetone (produced by the anal glands of the civet cat). (Interestingly, women who have had their ovaries removed are 100 to 1000 times less sensitive to these smells, suggesting that the sex hormone oestrogen affects smell sensitivity.) Musk and civet have been used for hundreds of years in perfumes, and musk odours are chemically related to the male hormone testosterone. When androstenone, the musky-smelling steroid similar to that found in the sweat and urine of men, was sprayed on a seat in a doctor's waiting room, women seemed attracted to the chair. Experiments with spraying telephones at a London train station produced similar results.

Smell activates the oldest and deepest parts of our brain, the limbic system. It's no coincidence that most of the world's religions use incense to induce an ecstatic, emotional state of consciousness, making the faithful more susceptible to the ritual and religious rites. Brain scans of people in prayer and meditation have shown that during intense religious experiences the limbic system becomes unusually active. Neurosurgeons who stimulate the limbic system during open-brain surgery say that patients occasionally report experiencing religious sensations. Studies of the ingredients of incense show that there is a relationship between the scents they give off and the scents of the human body: 'Suffice to say that the inspiration men get from incense is that it stimulates them in a truly profound manner, unconsciously stirring vestigial memory traces associated with times when odorous sex attractants played a vital role in the preservation of the species,' writes Stoddart.

Smell acts on us before we have time to think. A scent can ambush us, conjuring up memories and images in an instant. Walking down a city street, I get a whiff of a kretek, a clove cigarette, and am transported instantly to Indonesia, with its dusty roads and rickety food stalls lit with kerosene lamps. Proust was famously waylaid by a tea-soaked Madeleine. As he wrote: 'When nothing else from the past subsists, after people are dead, after the destruction of things, smell and taste alone remain, like souls bearing resiliently, on tiny and almost impalpable drops of their essence, the vast edifice of memory.'

Smell and taste, of course, are inseparable. We can taste only four flavours: sweet, sour, salty, bitter. According to Dr Alan Hirsch of the Smell and Taste Treatment and Research Foundation, 90 per cent of taste is smell. 'This can be easily demonstrated by holding your nose and eating a chocolate bar. The taste of the chocolate will be similar to chalk.' Dr Hirsch, a neurologist and psychiatrist who sees himself as 'the Magellan of the nasal passages' has come up with many unusual research findings. For example, the combined odour of lavender and pumpkin pie increases penile blood flow by 40 per cent. Floral and spice odours significantly reduce the perception of a woman's weight by 1.86 kg (4.1 lb). 'More remarkably those men who found the floral and spice odour to be pleasant perceived the woman to be a full 5.45 kg [12 lb] less than her actual weight.' Dr Hirsch's research also found that the scent of grapefruit can cause men to perceive women to be an average of six years younger than they actually are. Good reasons to make sure your man keeps his nose clean.

THREE

Talk to the Hand

For 14 years New Zealander Clint Hallam lived without a right hand. Then one morning in 1998 he woke up and there it was again. Of course, it wasn't the hand he was born with. His was the first successful transplanted hand from a cadaver. For many people it would be disconcerting to have a dead stranger's hand put breakfast toast into one's mouth or pick one's nose or perform the myriad intimate tasks a right hand is called upon to do. There are other considerations too. A hand transplant means your chances of getting an accurate reading from your palmist is reduced by 50 per cent. And if you're an ex-con like Hallam, the police are not going to be too happy about having their fingerprint records mucked up. As it turned out, Hallam and his hand didn't get on. In 2001 he rejected it before it rejected him: in short he had it cut off. Successful hand transplants, though, continue to be performed; the number, to use a handy expression, has now reached double digits.

Contemplating my hands at many a boring meeting, I've often thought a new hand would be difficult to turn down. As well as being the chief organ of our fifth sense, touch, the hand is an engineering marvel. Our unique ability to join thumb and forefinger is responsible for our technological advance over every other creature. As Professor John Napier wrote in his classic study, *Hands*: 'One cannot emphasize enough the importance of finger thumb opposition for human emergence from a relatively undistinguished primate background. Through natural selection, it promoted the adoption of upright posture and bipedal walking, tool using and tool making that, in turn, led to an enlargement of the brain through a positive feedback mechanism. In a sense it was probably the single most adaptation in our evolutionary history.' (Unfortunately, evolutionary adaptation of the hand never reckoned with shrink-wrapped food: for that we are thrown back on our Neanderthal skills of ripping prey apart with our teeth.)

Hands hold many clues to our physical, emotional and mental states as well as to our social status – a fact that palmists rely on to guide their readings. A simian crease, for example, which runs right across the upper palm (instead of the three creases most people have) is associated with conditions such as Down's syndrome, foetal alcohol syndrome and Aarskog syndrome. (Then again you could be like Tony Blair and Charles Manson or the one in 30 otherwise healthy people who have this abnormality.) If the palms of your hands are unusually red, it could mean cirrhosis of the liver or hypertension. If you are a smoker and your hands are usually icy cold, it may be that smoking is constricting blood vessels in the extremities and damaging your body. Normally, the hand should be comfortably warm.

Fingernails can offer many clues to your general health. Do you have Beau's lines – indentations that run across the nail? This happens when growth at the nail root is interrupted by severe illness such as heart attack or pneumonia. Vertical ridges that run the length of your nails become more obvious as you age and may accompany kidney failure. A condition called clubbing where the fingertips widen and become round may indicate heart disease or cancer. Lung disease is present in 80 per cent of people who have clubbed fingers. Yellow nail syndrome – one or two turn yellow or green and the cuticle or the moon disappears – is linked with respiratory diseases such as chronic bronchitis. Terry's nails – opaque and white nails with a dark pink to brown band at the nail tip – is sometimes associated with cirrhosis, congestive heart failure, adult-onset diabetes, cancer or ageing.

Over 70 medical conditions may manifest themselves in the hand. Hand examination, you'd think, would be a part of every doctor's diagnostic repertoire, yet the only reason I've ever been required to take my hand out of my pocket when I've consulted a doctor has been to extract my wallet. Some recent research even suggests that it may be possible not only to predict the onset of certain conditions such as heart disease and depression from little more than a cursory glance at fingers, but also such traits as musical aptitude, sporting prowess and sexual inclination.

Fingers have long been regarded as important body parts. Unlike toes, they have all been given names. The naming of the digits has been traced back to the laws of compensation for the loss of fingers and thumbs in Britain in AD 616. The *auricularis* or little finger got its name because it was the one most commonly used for extracting wax from ears. There's no need to point out the meaning of *demonstratorius* (index finger). *Impudicus* was the name for the middle finger, proof that humans have been giving each other the finger for well over a millennium, and *annualaris* was the ring finger. The ring finger was also once known as *medicus*, so named, it's said, because physicians used that digit to stir their nostrums.

The length of our fingers is determined by hormones, especially testosterone, in the first trimester of pregnancy – and the finger length ratio never changes as we grow to adulthood. Our fingers, then, are a marker for early foetal development, a critical stage in the growth of brain and body. This fact intrigued Dr John Manning, a biologist at the University of Liverpool, whose research has determined that finger length could be a significant indicator of bodily health and personal characteristics. Typically, Manning's research shows men's ring fingers are longer than their index fingers, while women's index and ring fingers tend to be the same length. Why? Because males are exposed to greater amounts of testosterone in the womb. The ratio of the index finger length to the ring length is called the 2D:4D digit ratio. In the average Caucasian male the ring finger is about 2 per cent longer than the index finger.

Interesting patterns start to appear when you relate these findings to real people. Manning and his colleagues examined 151 heart attack victims in the Liverpool area. They found that in men with relatively long index fingers, the age range for heart attack was 35 to 80 years of age. In those with relatively long ring fingers it was 58 to 80. An explanation for this difference is that men with long ring fingers have higher levels of testosterone, known to protect against heart attacks. Manning's findings, if confirmed by other studies, would mean that the length of a boy's ring finger could indicate if they have a higher risk of heart attack in early adulthood.

Manning and others have also found correlations between ring-finger length and depression in men and people with autism. A study of 102 men and women from different socio-economic backgrounds found that men with long digits, particularly ring fingers scored highest on the Beck Depression Inventory (BDI), a widely used means of detecting depression. Testosterone has long been associated with depression but the mechanism is not understood.

Manning has also studied the hands of autistic children and found that they have extremely long ring fingers compared to their index fingers (children with Asperger's syndrome also have abnormal digit ratios but less so). The finding supports the 'extreme male brain' theory of autism; that is, problems with communication and empathy, characteristic of men, become magnified in the autistic.

The significance of long ring fingers is not confined to negative traits. Manning has also found a strong correlation between long ring fingers and sporting ability. The more testosterone you have the better your spatial judgement, an important ability in many sports. A study of athletics and soccer showed that success was associated with long ring fingers. Professional footballers, for example, had longer ring fingers than non-football players; international footballers had longer ring fingers than non-international footballers; and 'stars' and coaches had longer ring fingers than current players, particularly those from lower divisions.

Because of their greater foetal exposure to testosterone, men with long ring fingers, Manning says, may be more fertile, more aggressive and assertive, have a greater proclivity towards homosexuality/bisexuality, and have more aptitude for music. Women who have relatively long ring fingers also share a greater tendency towards homosexuality/ bisexuality, are more aggressive and less fertile than those women with second and fourth digits of similar length.

Other research is starting to support Manning's hypothesis. A study by researchers at Monash University in Melbourne found that women with polycystic ovary syndrome (PCOS), an hormonal disorder that can cause, among other things, irregular menstrual periods, have finger length patterns similar to men.

In an attempt to debunk the hypothesis Professor Tim Spector, of the Twin Research Unit at St Thomas' Hospital, London, examined x-rays of the hands of 607 female twins aged 25 to 79 from his database and compared the lengths of the their index and ring fingers. To his surprise, the results, which he reported in the *British Journal of Sports Medicine*, showed women with longer ring fingers were significantly better at most sports, especially those involving running, such as tennis and soccer.

In some ways the idea of a correlation between finger length and traits such as autism, homosexuality and sporting ability is reminiscent of phrenology, the theory that aspects of character, personality and criminality could be determined by measuring bumps on the head. Phrenology was wildly popular in the 19th century, but is rightly regarded now as pseudoscience.

Manning has described the evidence for his hypothesis as persuasive but not yet definitive. It's also worth remembering that there is substantial overlap between the sexes; some men will have digit ratios typical of women and vice versa, just as some women are taller than some men. Environmental factors can also override inborn traits. Still, it could be a worry how much your hands reveal about you. It may be prudent to keep them out of sight at a job interview or on a first date. Unless, of course, they're not your own.

FOUR

Don't Torture Your Soles

One of the saddest museum exhibits I ever saw was a pair of embroidered silk shoes worn by a Chinese woman last century. The shoes were so tiny they would scarcely have fit a six-year-old child. Small feet have long been regarded in China and elsewhere as a sign of good breeding and grace. At the age of five or six, the insteps of many Chinese girls were broken and the feet tightly bandaged. The four small toes were bent under the ball of the foot, with only the big toe left free for walking and balance. Gradually the foot became deformed, with the heel and toes brought as close as possible, creating a high arch. The Lotus Foot, named because the resulting walk resembled the delicate swaying of the lotus, was regarded as the most erotic part of the female anatomy.

No woman today, of course, would allow their feet to be deformed for the sexual titillation of men – or would she? An X-ray of the Lotus Foot, in fact, resembles the X-ray of a woman in high heels. High heels force the foot into an unnatural pointed shape in an effort to make the feet appear as small as possible. It can be too much of a squeeze for some. In New York some women are resorting to 'cosmetic toe amputation' to fit into their favourite high heels. However, according to writer and high-heel aficionado, J. J. Leganeur, the toe is not usually amputated. 'The toe [usually the second] is cut open, some bone removed and then . . . sewn back up. Then the tip of the toe shrinks. The procedure is similar to the way shrunken heads were made in the Amazon. The skull inside the head was removed, leaving only soft tissue.'

High heels increase female attractiveness by accentuating hip movement and creating an uneasy gait that makes women appear more vulnerable and men more masterful. In fifteenth-century Italy, aristocratic women tottered in shoes with heels of between 15 cm (6 in) and 45 cm (18 in). Chopines, as they were called, reached their peak at 76 cm (30 in) and a law was passed in Venice in 1430 prohibiting their use by pregnant women. Who would have thought, though, that in the 21st century women would still be pandering to male fantasies of female weakness? Even women who eschew high heels still hanker after dainty feet and squeeze them into ill-fitting shoes. By one estimate, over 80 per cent of women wear shoes that are too small for them.

It's hardly surprising when you remember that one of the classic stories of childhood is the tale of Cinderella whose small feet won her the heart of the prince. The story is a glorification of the small foot as a symbol of femininity and sexual desirability. The Cinderella story, an erotic folktale cleaned up for children by the Grimm brothers, has hundreds of versions throughout the world, dating back to ancient Egypt. In the original Grimm's tale, one stepsister cuts off a toe and the other a heel to be able to fit into Cinderella's glass slipper. It's believed that a ninth-century Chinese version of the Cinderella story gave rise to the custom of foot binding that has crippled countless women for nearly a thousand years.

Podiatrists say that many of the problems our feet cause us are self-inflicted. Shoes, not just high heels, can be a major cause of foot injury. The trouble is that our feet bear little resemblance to the symmetrical models used to manufacture shoes. No pair of feet is identical – indeed no two feet are the same: the left foot is usually slightly larger than the right in right-handed people and vice versa. In two out of every ten people, the second toe is the longest one.

As Socrates observed, when our feet hurt we hurt all over. Because the 'foot bone's [actually there are 28 bones in each foot] connected to the leg bone and the leg bone's connected to the thigh bone' a pain in the foot can literally be a pain in the butt. The trauma caused by a foot problem will travel up the leg to the knee, hip and back. A blister from a new pair of shoes may be a minor irritation, but the resulting limp will upset the body's equilibrium. With every part of our body thrown off-balance, muscles will be put under extra strain and start to ache.

That's not to say reflexology, which claims that our feet are a microcosmic mirror of the total bodily system, has any scientific basis. If that were the case we might end up brain-damaged from an ingrown toenail or be asphyxiated by our bunions. However, in at least one case, a pain in the foot may point to a problem elsewhere. A painful Achilles tendon pain that lasts three days or more may be linked to heterozygous familial hypercholesterolaemia or HeFH, a genetic condition that carries a high risk of heart disease. A British study suggests that Achilles tendon pain lasting three days or more is 6.75 times more likely to occur in patients with HeFH than in the general population.

There's only one in a million chance you have HeFH, though. Foot problems in general are just that – localised, painful conditions that have plagued people from antiquity. BC does not stand for Before Corns. Corns were so prevalent in Hippocrates' time that he invented skin scrapers to pare them (an invention that was the forerunner of the scalpel). By the 17th century you could earn a living as a corn-cutter if you combined it with other services such as tooth-pulling. 'Corns cut very nicely' was part of London street peddlers' cries.

Corns, which are the direct result of wearing ill-fitting shoes, occur when the skin finds itself squeezed between the shoe on the outside and the foot on the inside. Often balloon-like sacs of fluid occur under the surface of the corn to cushion the underlying bones. Everything has been tried as a remedy for painful corns, from pastes made of swine dung or garden leeks to soaking in the gastric juices of animals. Onions in vinegar was once a popular cure. Urinating into your shoes was found to be a good way of softening both corn and leather. Corns are an excellent – but painful – way of predicting the weather. As atmospheric pressure drops, the fluid in the sacs beneath the corn expands, making it even more painful.

Bunions, another side effect of ill-fitting shoes, appear to run in families, though the exact role of heredity is not understood. Continuing year after year to squeeze your feet into pointed-toe shoes is a major risk factor (but flip flops or Jandals are not the answer because people scrunch their toes into a claw, causing tendonitis and even shin splints). Once the bunion has developed it will be impossible to get any shoe to fit well. There are, apparently, more than 100 different surgical procedures to correct bunions. But like warts, bunions are not something many want to admit to having. Instead of saying 'I'm having my bunions done', say, 'Actually it's my *hallux valgus*, if you must know ...' and people will be too embarrassed to inquire further.

Fungus foot (*tinea pedis*) was a mite embarrassing too until a public relations firm dreamed up the name 'athlete's foot' after a campaign to sell anti-fungal medication for 'policeman's foot' failed to generate sales. Athlete's foot has more to do with foot hygiene than athletics. Even the most dedicated couch potato can get it: all that's required is the creation of a warm, moist, dark environment in which fungi thrive. Wearing dry shoes, sprinkling cornstarch inside shoes before and after wearing, washing feet thoroughly at least twice a day, changing socks at least twice a day (cotton ones are best for absorbing moisture) will go a long way towards preventing athlete's foot.

The same dry environment will help prevent bromhidrosis, better known to the nose as smelly feet. One of the main causes of smelly feet is the presence of fetid bacteria between the toes. When we sweat, the fatty acids that we excrete decompose, creating an even fouler smell. Nervous tension or stress produces sweat which, unlike normal healthy perspiration, has its own unpleasant odour – the smell of fear. Strong foods like garlic and onion can taint the smell of ordinary sweat and increase the foul smell of feet. Another cause of smelly feet is foot fatigue, which can cause the feet to sweat excessively. A nervous disease or a blood disorder like anaemia can also cause foot odour.

Flat feet are nothing to worry about or seek treatment for, though they were once considered unlucky and a sign of evil. In the Middle Ages, flat feet was one of the signs you were a witch. In the 19th century, flat feet was given the medical term 'Jewish foot', a condition that became synonymous with lazy and useless. By the less anti-Semitic 20th century the condition became known as weak foot, and only men with an arch in their foot were selected to serve in the army. Ironically, studies show that people with flat feet are usually fast runners and are less likely to become injured.

Not all foot conditions are aptly named. Few car-bound police officers, today, would probably suffer from policeman's heel caused by standing or walking for long periods on hard surfaces like concrete. Policeman's heel, also known as calcaneal bursitis, is caused by an inflammation of a bursa just under the weight-bearing surface of the heel bone. One home treatment is to pad the heel, cutting a hole in the pad so no pressure is placed on the inflamed bursa. Soaking feet in a solution of Epsom salts and hot water for an hour also helps. For chronic sufferers the painful bursa may be removed with surgery.

Policeman's heel can affect a whole range of workers from posties and assembly-line workers to waiters. Waiters not only have to worry about their heels but also their toes. In cafés and restaurants, waiters carrying dishes in both hands rely on their toes to kick open the kitchen door. Doing this day after day this can lead to chronic inflammation of the inner side of the big toe. It can also cause an ingrown toenail and in time a corn may develop beneath the nail. Here's a tip for your waiter: don't kick the door.

FIVE

Keep in Touch

There's a deep irony in the fact that we have never been more connected and never more out of touch. Cell phones and email make us contactable at any time or place but reduce the likelihood of physical encounters. And the more we use technology to communicate, the shyer we are likely to become about reaching out and touching someone. Faith Popcorn, dubbed the Nostradamus of marketing by *Fortune* magazine, predicts that our hunger for human touch will soon become a target for commercial exploitation. Airlines, she says, may hire actors to greet you with a hug, and financial advisers may literally hold your hand through tough times. Phone booths will be replaced by mechanised hugging booths. And why not caressing ATMs? (You're more than a PIN to us.)

It would be a shame if touch became another technique to manipulate our emotions. Until now it has been our most reliable, trustworthy sense. In the *Bible*, the apostle Thomas refuses to believe the story of the resurrection until he has touched the lance wound in Christ's side. As Margaret Atwood says in *The Blind Assassin*, 'Touch comes before sight, before speech. It is the first language and the last, and it always tells the truth.' It's also the most intimate sense: when you feel something it is right next to your body. In *Nineteen Eighty-Four*, George Orwell's nightmarish vision of a totalitarian all-seeing state, Winston Smith, unable to look at his lover Julia without betraying her, surreptitiously touches her, learning 'every detail of her hand'.

For children, human touch is close to magic. Premature infants massaged for 15 minutes three times a day gained weight 47 per cent faster than those who were left alone in incubators. Babies communicate through their bodies; touch signals to them that they are safe. Lack of touch can cause brain damage and death in many instances. This has been known since the 13th century. In a bizarre test, Frederick II, the last Emperor of the Holy Roman Empire, devised an experiment to find out what language children would speak if they had never been spoken to. He separated a group of newborns from their mothers and had them raised by nurses who provided food and shelter for the children without speaking to them. Deprived of human interaction, all the children died. Frederick, observed one thirteenth-century historian had 'laboured in vain ... for they could not live without the petting'.

The lesson, however, was not learned by succeeding generations. Up until the second decade of the 20th century, the death rate for children under the age of one in American institutions was nearly 100 per cent. They died of infantile atrophy or marasamus, (Greek for wasting away). Lack of loving human attention also manifested itself in children adopted from Romanian orphanages in the 1980s. Many of the children spent months or years lying for up to 20 hours a day in their cots. Canadian researcher Elinor Ames tracked the progress of children who had been adopted by Canadian families. Compared with non-adopted Canadian children and

Romanian children adopted before the age of four months who had never lived in an institution, the Romanian orphanage children had lower IQs, more behaviourial problems, and at 10 years old were still showing what the study called 'atypical insecure patterns'.

Studies with animals confirm the importance of touch in early life. Neurologist Dr Saul Schanberg showed that when laboratory pup rats were licked by the mother rat it slowed the pup rat production of beta-endorphin, a chemical that affects the levels of insulin and growth hormone.

Researchers were able to produce the same effect by using a wet paintbrush to stimulate the stroke of the mother's tongue. Schanberg has speculated that touch is part of a primitive survival mechanism found in all mammals, including humans. Slowing metabolism through the mother's touch gives the infant a better chance of survival while the mother is away by decreasing the need for food. However, if the absence is prolonged, growth is stunted. Children who live in emotionally dysfunctional families may become stunted, a condition that even growth hormones won't remedy. Children who have not experienced much physical contact can become hypersensitive to touch. One child adopted from a Romanian orphanage could not stand the sensation of walking barefoot for the first two years.

In his book *Touching: The Human Significance of the Skin*, anthropologist Ashley Montagu argues that 'The tactually failed child grows into an individual who is not only physically awkward in his relations with others, but who is psychologically, behaviourally awkward with them. Such persons are likely to be found wanting in that tact which the Oxford Dictionary defines as "the ready and delicate sense of what is fitting and proper in dealing with others ... There appears to be a very distinct carry over from tactile experience in infancy to tactful experience in later life.' Boys who don't get enough tactile affection grow into men who almost crush the hands they shake and who display affection to their friends by punching them in the chest or abdomen.

But, outside of lovemaking, how essential is touching for adults? Apes and monkeys, our closest relatives, spend up to a fifth of each day grooming or being groomed by other group members. As psychologist Robin Dunbar says in his book *Grooming, Gossip, and the Evolution of Language*, grooming is not just a matter of hygiene but a way of cementing bonds, making friends and influencing fellow primates. But in humans, Dunbar argues, language evolved to replace social grooming because the grooming time required by our large groups made impossible demands on our time. 'Language ... evolved to fill the gap because it allows us to use the time available for social interaction more efficiently.'

Cell phones allow us to groom each other from afar and help us bond. But touch still remains important, says Dunbar, because words are completely inadequate at the emotional level. 'When the relationship reaches the point of greatest intensity, we abandon language and return to the age-old rituals of mutual mauling and direct stimulation. At this crucial point in our lives, grooming – of all the things we inherit from our primate ancestry – resurfaces as the way to reinforce our bonds. We use it because physical contact is deeply moving and reassuring in a way language cannot be. And it achieves that because monotonous stroking and rubbing stimulates opiate production much more effectively than words can ever do.'

When we are touched in a loving way, it increases the levels of the hormone oxytocin. Sometimes called the cuddle hormone, oxytocin has been shown to calm the body and promote social bonding and trust between people. Orgasm achieved through sex with a partner produces the biggest oxytocin hit. In one study comparing couples who engaged in penetrative sex, non-coital sex, masturbation or abstinence, psychologist Stuart Brody of the University of Paisley found that the couples who had penetrative sex had the lowest blood pressure when undergoing stressful tests of public speaking and doing mental arithmetic out loud. The calming effects lasted for up to a week. Those who abstained had the highest blood pressure response to stress. (It's intriguing that self-touch can result in orgasm but self-tickling is impossible. The porn industry should thank God it's not the other way around.)

There is evidence that oxytocin levels can also increase through massage. The Touch Research Institute at the University of Miami School of Medicine has conducted many studies that show the benefit of massage, especially for many different kinds of pain. The Institute has found massage to be effective in relieving chronic pain in arthritis and diabetes, and useful in treating eating disorders, chronic fatigue, fibromyalgia and HIV-associated diseases. 'We have looked at the A-to-Z of medical conditions, and we have not found a single condition massage has not been effective for,' the Institute's Director, Tiffany Field, has said.

Not everybody wants to be touched, though, and there are touching taboos in most cultures. There's an irony that we are quick to pat or stroke pets but are apprehensive about touching other human beings. Touching can also be a status gesture, as Diane Ackerman noted in her book, *A Natural History of the Senses*: 'Researchers observing hundreds of people in public settings in a small town in Indiana and in a big city on the East

Coast, found that males touch females first, that females are more likely to touch females than males are to touch males, and that people of higher status generally touch lower-status people first. Lower-status people wait for the go ahead before they risk an increased intimacy – even a subconscious one – with their presumed superiors.'

Whether we benefit from being touched may depend on our own physiological make-up – and our gender. A study by researchers at the University of North Carolina School of Medicine found that caressing a woman in a non-sexual way can have the same effect on her blood pressure as blood-pressure-lowering medication. However, stroking had no perceptible effect on men's blood pressure. The researchers speculate that testosterone blunted the effect of any increase in oxytocin.

When we touch someone or something we experience our body, our place in the physical world. 'Touch teaches us that life has depth and contour; it makes our sense of the world and our self three-dimensional. Without that intricate feel for life there would be no artists, whose cunning is to make sensory and emotional maps, and no surgeons, who dive through the body with their fingers,' writes Diane Ackerman.

It's possible, however, to go for days or even weeks without touching someone. Touch deprivation causes us to feel isolated, depressed and hypersensitive to touch. A casual brush of skin may seem like an electric shock. 'The electricity that is often, metaphorically speaking, said to pass between people when touching one another may be something more than a mere metaphor,' writes Ashley Montagu. 'The skin is an especially good electrical conductor ... Electrical changes acting through the automatic nervous system produce an increase in electrical conductance of the skin (a decrease in resistance) across the palms of the hands or feet. There can be little doubt that in tactile stimulation electrical changes are transmitted from one individual to the other.'

Has our increasing use of technology to communicate and the sexualisation of touching made us more touch-deprived than previous generations? It's hard to be sure but certainly we live in a culture where touching, mainly in a sexual context, is seen as a highly desirable, not to say essential, part of a fulfilling life. Touching, the message goes, is part of a healthy lifestyle and we become anxious if we are not getting enough. In New York, two entrepreneurial relationship counsellors, Reid Mihalko and Marcia Baczynski, have spotted a gap in the market and set up Cuddle Parties, social events where adults in pyjamas pay $30 to get physically close to others. No sex is allowed in these 'boundary appropriate workshops' and a trained 'Cuddle Lifeguard' is always on duty to discourage dry humping or worse. Could Cuddles replace Tupperware as a suburban social event?

Perhaps the beneficial effects of touch will be sold to us in a bottle. In 1955, biochemist Vincent du Vigneaud won the Nobel Prize in Chemistry for synthesising oxytocin. Synthetic oxytocin, also called Pitocin or Syntocinon, is used primarily to bring on contractions in pregnant women and sometimes to release the milk for breastfeeding. However, some intriguing uses for synthetic oxytocin have come to light. Researchers at the University of Zurich have discovered that when oxytocin is administered by a nasal spray it can promote trust between people, even to the point where they are prepared to part with money. In a game involving an 'investor' and an 'anonymous trustee', those who were sprayed with oxytocin invested 17 per cent more money with those they had never met before than the investors who had been sprayed with a placebo. Drug companies are already developing oxytocin-based drugs that could be used in psychotherapy and the treatment of mental conditions, from crippling shyness to autism and schizophrenia. 'Social Viagra', as one researcher called oxytocin, could also become a lifestyle drug to ease those stressful situations such as public speaking or party mingling.

Touch is so powerful that it affects us even when we are unconsciously aware of it. For example, experiments have shown that vocational counsellors who touched their clients during a counselling session were rated as more expert than those who did not touch. Students who were 'accidentally' touched by librarians when their library cards were being returned gave the librarians and the library a higher rating than did a control group of students. Researchers have also found that diners who had been touched on the hand or shoulder by a waitress tipped better than those who had not been touched at all. The tips got higher when the waitress touched the female in a male–female couple. Women, it seems, are a soft touch.

SIX

Obsess About Oral Hygiene

The only people who remember my birthday with any consistency are the local video store owner and my dentist. From the video store I get a card that can be exchanged for a free video, and from my dentist a 10 per cent discount coupon on my next visit. Invariably I use the former and bin the latter: going to the dentist hardly qualifies as a birthday treat. Like most people, though, I feel guilty about not going more regularly. When you're in your twenties you can probably get away with not going to the dentist too often. By the time you hit middle age, avoiding regular check-ups can have dire consequences. If not treated, periodontal disease, caused by the accumulation of bacteria and plaque, can progress to the point where the only solution is to yank the teeth out.

It's easy to get complacent about oral hygiene – that's because the facts of oral ecology are rarely spelled out as precisely as Dr Mel Rosenberg did in a *Scientific American* article: 'At any given time, oral bacteria, usually anaerobic, may be producing hydrogen sulfide, with its distinctive rotten-egg smell; methyl mercaptan and skatole, also present in faeces; indole, used in small amounts in perfume but foul in large quantities; cadaverine, associated with rotting corpses;

putrescine, found in decaying meat; and isovaleric acid, which smells like sweaty feet. No wonder human breath can at times be so offensive.'

More than 615 different species of micro-organisms, mostly bacteria, live in the mouth of every adult. In one mouth the number of bacteria can easily exceed the number of people who live on earth. Billions of them grow in layers, inhabit every moist nook and cranny, every slimy surface. With an average temperature of 95° and a saliva-induced humidity of 100 per cent, it's a perfect breeding environment. Brush your teeth regularly and bacteria that live on each tooth surface may be contained at anything between 1000 and 100,000. If you don't have a particularly clean mouth it's likely you have 100 million to 1 billion bacteria growing on *each* tooth. Introduce sugar or a simple carbohydrate into your gob and bacteria go on a feeding frenzy, producing acid that will eventually eat through the enamel of your teeth. By the time you feel toothache, the acids will have eaten through to the tooth's underlying dentin and pulp layers where the nerves are located.

It's not just our teeth that are at risk. Oral bacteria can affect the heart when they enter the bloodstream. Scientists theorise that they may attach to fatty plaques in the coronary arteries and contribute to clot formation. Another theory is that the inflammation caused by periodontal disease increases plaque build-up in the arteries. Whatever the mechanism, studies have found that people with periodontal disease are twice as likely as those without it to suffer from coronary heart disease. It doesn't end there. If root infections in certain teeth in the upper jaw are not treated, the bacteria can spread to cause serious eye infections, even blindness. That's why they're called eye teeth. Some diseased upper-jaw teeth can spread infection to nerves and blood vessels of the face and to the veins leading to the brain. If a tooth in the lower jaw is badly diseased, the bacteria may travel to the throat and cause a rare condition known as Ludwig's angina in which the larynx swells so much that it's impossible to breathe.

Tooth decay only became endemic in the early 1800s with the widespread cultivation of sugar beet. Until William Addis invented the modern toothbrush during a stay in England's Newgate Prison in 1770, most people cleaned their teeth with rags. In the 18th century, laughing was considered extremely bad manners in polite society, partly because it displayed a great many rotting stumps of teeth and expelled foul odours.

As Elizabeth Burton says in *The Georgians At Home*, fans were a godsend for the orthodontically challenged. 'Apart from the normal fanning and flirtatious function, it could be used to hide a smile which displayed a squalid lot of teeth or as a screen to protect the nose against mephitic breath.' Breath fresheners and perfumes were wildly overused. 'The unpalatable truth is that without the liberal use of civet, musk, ambergris and various strong essences no room full of people was likely to be habitable for long,' writes Burton. Unfortunately by the time Oscar Wilde came along, fans for men were out of fashion, and he had to dispense his best witticisms from behind his hand because his teeth had been turned black by mercury treatment for syphilis.

Not all the bacteria in your mouth rots your teeth. Some produce organic acids such as proprionic and buteric acid, which kill organisms that can cause intestinal problems. The bacteria responsible for most tooth decay, *Streptococcus mutans*, arrive with our baby teeth. They're kindly passed on by parents spewing saliva as they coo into the face of the child whose teeth are emerging. (Human babies are born with sterile mouths, but within minutes to hours their mouths are colonised with bacteria and other organisms that stay with them until they die.)

Saliva helps to protect against some of the bacterial effects by neutralising acid, killing some bacteria and causing other bacteria to clump together so that they don't adhere to teeth and are washed away. Radiation treatment for head or neck cancer as well as many medications can have a serious effect on our dental health. They cause a huge drop in saliva production and allow bacteria to run rampant. Sleeping also has its effect, too. As science writer Jane R. Stevens put it so lyrically: 'During a night's sleep when saliva production drops to near zero, bacteria, like the minions in the Fantasia version of Moussorgsky's "A Night on Bald Mountain" revel in their freedom and multiply with abandon until dawn.'

After a night playing host to cavorting bacteria, it's hardly surprising our mouths smell like a dumpster. And for many that smell never seems to go away. The world is divided into two camps: those who have halitosis and those who think they have it. The former, though, is greatly outnumbered by the latter. Though it's often assumed that bad breath is caused by gases rising from the stomach, the main source is the back of the tongue, which traps oral debris and gunk from postnasal drip that does not get washed away with saliva. Infected tonsils account for about 3 per cent of halitosis cases. Around 1 per cent can be a symptom of hundreds of other diseases from diabetes to lung disease. In 5 to 10 per cent of cases the smell is not coming from the mouth at all but from the nostrils, which can produce foul odours when the flow of mucus is impeded by conditions such as sinusitis.

Imaginary bad breath, though, may be more of a problem.

Over decades we've been conditioned by advertising to believe we don't do nearly enough to avoid offending others with our smells. Listerine, for example, has been around for more than a century (as a regular Listerine-swiller I wasn't surprised to learn it was once sold as a floor cleaner and a cure for gonorrhoea). In the 1920s, the company hit on a way to medicalise bad breath by calling it halitosis and, with advertising slogans such as 'Even your best friends won't tell you' and 'Always a bridesmaid never a bride', sales took off. The company's revenues rose from $115,000 to more than $8 million in just seven years. Along the way it also created a new psychological condition: halitophobia.

This secret fear of halitosis apparently now affects millions. Most halitophobics obsess about oral hygiene but manage to get on with their lives. The most desperate endlessly consult specialists, socially isolate themselves, have all their teeth extracted or even commit suicide. The sad irony is that, as studies show, those who are convinced they have bad breath usually have odour-free mouths, while those with halitosis are blissfully unaware of their own stink. To objectively test for bad breath, Dr Rosenberg suggests carefully scraping the back of the tongue with a spoon. If there is yellowish mucus on the spoon take a sniff. 'The odour of this material on the spoon itself is often very reminiscent of the odour emanating from the whole mouth of the subject.'

It's hard to believe that most people, at least in the US, didn't brush their teeth every day until after World War II when returning soldiers introduced the army ritual into civilian life. Now brushing and flossing is regarded as essential to oral hygiene. As periodontist Dr Ruth Garcia told a dental research conference: 'Floss or die!' Tongue scraping may soon be de rigueur, though there's not much evidence to suggest that tongue scraping is much more effective in improving oral hygiene than ordinary brushing. And is there a case for banning kissing? Scientists now believe that *Porphyromonas gingivalis*, long suspected as the cause of serious gum disease, is contagious and can be transmitted by kissing. In the parallel universe of micro-organisms, a kiss is never just a kiss.

SEVEN

Just Walk

It's a reflection of our times that the simple pleasure of walking has become unaffordable for many people. Walking, they feel, is beyond their means: they are time-poor. However, from another perspective it is cheap health insurance. Walking may reduce the risk of heart disease, breast cancer, diabetes, colon cancer and stroke. A brisk three-kilometre walk can reduce the risk of impotence by improving blood flow through the blood vessels. Jogging may get you fitter more quickly, but causes wear and tear on the joints. No pain no gain is a masochist's lie. Research shows that moderate exercise can be just as beneficial as the more vigorous sort. You can lose weight even with short daily walks. By walking just 10 minutes twice a day you can reduce your body weight by 10 per cent over 18 months. That makes walking just as effective in losing weight as with some diet pills. In one study, for example, people taking three Xenical (orlistat) a day lose an average of only 6 kg (12 lb) after two years. Unlike walkers, Xenical pill-poppers may also have to put up with side effects like flatulence and faecal incontinence.

But walking has benefits beyond weight loss and the prevention of physical illness – it promotes a feeling of well-being and puts us in touch with things that can easily become overlooked in the hurly-burly of daily life. At a simple level, walking relieves stress and helps lift depression. Walking connects us with the world and our own bodies, connections that are becoming increasingly eroded by technology. As the historian G. M. Trevelyan puts it: 'I have two doctors, my left leg and my right. When body and mind are out of gear (and those twin parts of me live at such close quarters that one always catches the melancholy from the other), I know I shall only have to call in my doctors and I shall be well again.' Recent studies confirm Trevelyan's observation. A US study, for example, found that in adults aged 20 to 45 with mild to moderate depression, 30-minute aerobic sessions three to five times a week reduced depressive symptoms by almost 50 per cent. That is similar to treatment with antidepressant medication.

Walking is exercise that you can take at your own pace and in your own time. Three 10-minute brisk walks five days a week can increase fitness as much as walking continuously for 30 minutes over the same period, one study found. Including a steep hill on your walk will increase your aerobic fitness by boosting your heart rate by about 20 per cent. Beach walking can make you work harder because the sand absorbs the downward motion of each step and you need more energy to lift your foot again. Walking in soft snow is three times more demanding than walking on the pavement. Retro walking or walking backwards consumes 25 per cent more calories, but you'll need wing mirrors and an indifference to the stares and chuckles of passers-by.

Walking is such a low-tech mundane activity that it can be hard to get motivated to make it a daily practice despite the evidence that it will do us a world of good. The very word 'pedestrian' is synonymous with 'unexciting', 'humdrum'. As well, most of us live in suburbs that make for dull walks, an endless procession of undistinguished houses and garages set among uniform squares of lawn. A book that got me off the couch was Rebecca Solnit's fascinating *Wanderlust: A History of Walking*. As Solnit points out, walking or bipedality, is the defining characteristic of human development. 'Walking,' says Solnit, 'is a state in which the mind, the body and the world are aligned, as though there were three characters finally in conversation together, three notes suddenly making a chord. Walking allows us to be in our bodies and in the world without being made busy by them. It leaves us free to think without being wholly lost in our thoughts.'

We now live, she argues, in a series of interiors – home, car, gym, office, shops – disconnected from each other. 'On foot everything stays connected, for while walking one occupies the spaces between these interiors in the same way one occupies the interiors. One lives in the whole world rather than in interiors built up against it.'

When we walk we are taking part in a great human tradition. The Greek philosophers were known as the Peripatetic School – the word peripatetic means 'one who walks habitually and extensively'. For many, walking has been a great aid to thought – and has been practised by philosophers from Jean-Jacques Rousseau to Thomas Hobbes, who had an ink-horn built into his walking stick so that he could jot down notes as he went along.

Poet William Wordsworth was one of history's great walkers, having 'traversed a distance of 175 to 180,000 English miles' according to Thomas De Quincey. Wordsworth composed poetry as he walked – the rhythm of his walking can be detected in one of his best poems 'Tintern Abbey'.

When we walk we often fall into a reverie. James Joyce and Virginia Wolfe turned it into a literary device, the stream of consciousness famously used in *Ulysses* and *Mrs Dalloway*.

It's no longer possible to walk everywhere we need to go, even if we had the time. In countries like the US, walkers are regarded with suspicion in some areas, or their activities are hampered by a lack of pavements or by six-lane highways. 'In a sense the car has become a prosthetic, and though prosthetics are usually for injured and missing limbs, the auto-prosthetic is for a conceptually impaired body or a body impaired by the creation of a world that is no longer human in scale,' writes Solnit.

Since our bodies are becoming less needed for work or travel, the body has begun to atrophy as both a muscular and sensory organism. 'The body that used to have the status of a work animal now has the status of a pet: it does not provide real transport, as a horse might have; instead the body is exercised as one might a dog,' writes Solnit.

In the 16th century, palaces and mansions often included long narrow rooms called galleries to permit indoor walking when the weather was bad (eventually the gallery became a place for displaying paintings). But now many people walk indoors even in summer, using treadmills. 'Sisyphean contraptions,' Solnit calls them, 'devices with which to go nowhere in places where there is no nowhere to go'.

Strangely, people are prepared to pay money to exercise their bodies in a gym, but are reluctant to walk any distance. The 'mental radius of how far they are willing to go on foot seems to be shrinking: in defining neighbourhoods and shopping districts, planners say it is a quarter of a mile, the distance that can be walked in five minutes'.

Walking may keep us healthy, but it is also a political

act and an affirmation of the value we place on living and connecting with the world at a human pace. As Solnit writes: 'An indicator species signifies the health of an ecosystem and its endangerment or diminishment can be an early warning sign of systemic trouble. Walking is an indicator species of various kinds of freedoms and pleasures: free time, free and alluring space and unhindered bodies.'

EIGHT

Sleep On It

I have never subscribed to the theory that time is uniform. It's nonsense to suggest, for instance, that 15 minutes spent waiting in the cold is really just a quarter of an hour, or that the hours we spend asleep are the same length as daylight ones. Immediately we close our eyes, time is concertinaed: no sooner have we got comfortable in bed than it's time to get up.

In the 21st century that feeling is becoming more pronounced. Just a century ago people were sleeping between 9 and 10 hours a night. The average today is 7.5 hours – and on weekdays many people sleep less than that. That 20 per cent reduction in sleep time has a cost. In America, where they keep statistics on everything, it's estimated that sleep deprivation costs $150 billion a year in higher stress and reduced workplace productivity. Lack of sleep has been cited as a factor in the *Challenger* space shuttle disaster, the Chernobyl nuclear reactor meltdown, and the *Exxon Valdez* oil spill. It is often a contributing factor in plane, train and car crashes. It's probably time sleep deprivation was made as socially unacceptable as drink-driving. Time, perhaps, for television campaigns with celebrities boasting about how much they got last night or random sleep tests where drivers are required to listen to parliamentary speeches without nodding off.

It's macho, of course, to let it be known that you can get by on four or five hours' sleep a night. Those who need more, it's implied, lack drive and ambition. According to most scientists, individual sleep needs vary from about 5 to 10 hours per night, but the average is 8 hours. The importance of sleep is underestimated. Research suggests sleep is fundamental to good health. Rats deprived of sleep die within two weeks. Lack of sleep can make you fat: your body finds it harder to process blood sugar and increases appetite by reducing the levels of the appetite-depressing hormone leptin. Studies suggest that sleeping less than five hours a night over a period of years will increase your risk of premature death, heart disease and diabetes. Sleep deprivation affects your immune system, lowering your resistance and infection.

It could also affect your moral judgement. According to a study by the Walter Reed Army Institute of Research, sleeplessness may slow down the brain's ability to integrate cognitive and emotional information, which is needed to address serious moral dilemmas. Experiments with army volunteers showed many changed their minds about what was morally acceptable when they'd been deprived of sleep for two days.

Getting enough sleep may soon join getting enough exercise as a major health anxiety. Each year, for example, in the US the National Sleep Foundation, which has ties to the makers of sleeping pills, promotes its National Sleep Awareness Week. A recent poll it conducted found that 75 per cent of adult respondents had frequent difficulty sleeping. Pharmaceutical companies are reportedly gearing up to promote insomnia as the next epidemic. But are we really getting insufficient sleep?

Sleep deprivation is often regarded as a modern phenomenon, a consequence of electric lighting and the 24-hour society that the technology eventually made possible. But in his paper 'Sleep We Have Lost: Pre-Industrial Slumber in the British Isles', historian A. Roger Ekirch writes that getting a good night's sleep was often just as difficult for generations that had no artificial lighting. Today, people imagine themselves to have a sleep problem if they have a regular period of wakefulness during the night. For earlier generations two periods of sleep was the norm. After going to bed between 9 and 10 p.m., sleepers awoke from their 'fyrste slepe' around midnight, talked, smoked emptied their bladders, visited neighbours, prayed or lay in the dark reflecting on their dreams. Eventually they fell into a second or 'morning sleep'.

The wakeful interval was also a favourite time for love-making, says Ekirch. 'Significantly for our understanding of early modern demography, segmented sleep may have enhanced a couple's ability to conceive children, since fertility might have benefited from an interlude of rest. In fact, the sixteenth-century French physician Laurent Joubert concluded that early morning intercourse enabled plowmen, artisans and other labourers to beget numerous children. Because exhaustion prevented workers from copulating upon first going to bed, intercourse occurred "after the first sleep" when "they have more enjoyment" and "do it better".'

Another benefit of biphasic sleep was that people were able to recall and savour their dreams. We have between 100,000 and 200,000 dreams in our lifetimes. Most vanish with the first shrill of the alarm clock or are lost in the morning rush. A period of wakefulness in the night allowed dreams to be captured and explored in the conscious mind. With few other distractions on offer, dream analysis was a popular past time, generating much discussion and brisk sales of dream books. Dreams provided an escape from the drudgery, fear and oppressiveness of everyday living, a source of guidance and sometimes erotic delight. In his *Diary*, Samuel Pepys reflected on his night-time tryst with Lady Castlemaine – 'the best that ever was dreamed . . . all the dalliance I desired with her.' However, says Ekirch, 'so suspicious of his visions was Pepys's wife that she took to feeling his penis while he slept for signs of an erection'. (In fact tumescence occurs in both sexes when we dream but has little to do with erotic fantasy.)

Though dreams have been taken seriously for millennia, it was only with the publication of Sigmund Freud's *The Interpretation of Dreams* in 1900 that science began to take dreams seriously. Then in 1953 a young PhD student in Chicago, Eugene Aserinsky, saw something nobody had ever noticed before: during sleep there are periods of rapid eye movement (REM), which he later found was correlated with increased brain activity. Something very intense is going on when we sleep; on an electroencephalogram (EEG) trace it looks very similar to wakefulness. Aserinsky's discovery had scientists scrambling to find out, and sleep and dreaming became a hot research area.

But in 1977 Harvard neuroscientists Allan Hobson and Robert McCarley came up with a physiological explanation for dreams that suggested that dream analysis was a complete waste of time. Studying sleeping cats, Hobson and McCarley discovered that during REM sleep, when most dreams occur, the brain stem was flooded with the neurotransmitter acetylcholine while the levels of other neurotransmitters norepinephrine and serotonin plummeted. This, they said, resulted in the random firing of neurons. A dream was, in effect, 'a tale told by an idiot, full of sound and fury, signifying nothing'. Freud might as well have spent his time analysing tea leaves.

However, in the late 1990s London neuropsychologist Mark Solms found that patients could dream perfectly well despite having damage to the brain stem, which switches REM sleep off and on. Solms argued that dreaming actually takes place in the ventromesial forebrain, a more sophisticated area where our desires and urges originate. Solms discovered that patients who had a prefrontal leucotomy, a common surgical procedure for mental illness in the 1950s and 1960s, reported loss of dreaming. It was turning out that Freud's theory of dreams might not be so far off the mark after all. With sophisticated technology like magnetic resonance imaging (MRI) and positron emission tomography (PET), scientists have now found that the most active areas during REM are the limbic system, which controls our emotions, and the visual cortex, while the prefrontal and parietal cortices, which help us to be rational and logical, are largely inactive (this may explain why New Agers are attracted to dreams).

Why we sleep and dream remain mysteries, but theories abound. One theory is that it's non-REM sleep that is important. Some scientists believe that in this period of neuron inactivity the body goes to work replenishing proteins, strengthening synapses and so on. The frantic activity that takes place in REM sleep every 90 minutes is a process of testing to ensure that everything is working before further restoration work is carried out. Since the brain is constantly pruning surplus cells by a process called apoptosis or programmed cell death, another theory goes that the activity that takes place during

REM sleep is the way neurons signal that they are healthy and not to be culled. Experiments seem to support this theory: baby rats deprived of 60 per cent of their normal REM sleep showed abnormal apoptosis.

But there may be more than repair work going on during sleep. REM sleep could be helping us develop 'procedural memory', enabling us to learn complex tasks. In one experiment volunteers were asked to play a simple video game that involved quickly pressing a corresponding button when one of six lights flashed. Unbeknown to volunteers, the seemingly random sequence of flashing lights was programmed to a complex set of rules. Next day, the volunteers were divided into three groups and retested. Those who had a good night's sleep showed huge improvement. However, volunteers who had been deprived of REM sleep showed no improvement. And the clincher – volunteers who were tested on a game where the sequence was totally random showed no improvement. Sleep hadn't helped because there was nothing to learn.

But the most interesting research findings are that dreaming can help us problem-solve and be more creative. This theory, espoused by the likes of Harvard neuroscientist Robert Stickgold, suggests that the high acetylcholine levels we know occur in REM sleep cause neurons to act in unusual ways. 'It's biased towards weak, non-obvious and potentially useful connections,' Stickgold told *New Scientist* magazine. So our sleeping brain may be able to find solutions that our waking brain cannot. It's still unclear how useful a therapist our night self is, but experiments show that trying to suppress something increases the chances we will dream about it. Ex-smokers, for example, often dream about smoking. Whether dreams are really 'the royal road to knowledge of the unconscious' as Freud thought has yet to be determined. Some scientists argue that they are no more than relatively straightforward reflections of our daily preoccupations or the internal processing of stressful situations.

Nevertheless, many people have reason to be glad they paid attention to their dreams. In a fascinating little book, *The Committee of Sleep: How Artists, Scientists, and Athletes Use Dreams for Creative Problem Solving – And How You Can Too*, Harvard psychologist Deirdre Barrett cites scores of examples of dream-inspired success. The melody of Paul McCartney's most successful song 'Yesterday' came from a dream. 'Twice I have transferred dreams to film exactly as I had dreamed them,' confided director Ingmar Bergman. Frederick Fellini, Orson Welles and Robert Altman have also made liberal use of their dreams in films. A medical experiment dreamed up by physiologist Otto Loewi helped him win a Nobel Prize. Golfer Jack Nicklaus improved his swing by dreaming about it. Problem-solving, says Barrett, often takes place in the hypnagogic state, which occurs immediately upon falling asleep or just before awakening.

Sleeping on our problems may not always solve them, but after a good night's sleep, the world always seems a better place to be.

Mind

I find, by experience, that
the mind and the body are
more than married, for they
are most intimately united;
and when one suffers,
the other sympathises.

LORD CHESTERFIELD
BRITISH STATESMAN (1694–1773)

NINE

Take Your Own Sweet Time

In 1959, cardiologists Meyer Friedman and Ray Rosenman first used the label 'Type A Personality' to describe the pathologically impatient male who is driving himself to a heart attack. '"How can I move faster, and do more and more things in less and less time?" is the question that never ceases to torment him.' Fast forward – and fast forward is the *only* way ahead now – to 2007. Type A is the norm, applicable not only to male executives, but also to teachers, clerks, factory hands, part-time working mothers, and even children.

In what has been called 'the everydayathon' of modern life, time seems to have contracted. Dr Larry Dossey, who coined the term 'hurry sickness', used to ask his patients to sit quietly in a chair and say when they thought a minute had elapsed. The record went to a manager who said 'That's a minute' after only nine seconds. Dossey believed that this common distortion of time is more than a psychological quirk. 'The perceptions of passing time that we observe from our external clocks cause our internal clocks to run faster.' In the long term, that may lead to heart disease, high blood pressure or depression of our immune function.

In our hyper world, even appliances struggle to keep up:

toasters come with 'extra fast browning facility', express irons heat up more quickly, answering machines play back 25 per cent faster. DVD software now allows you to speed up movies without a chipmunk effect on the soundtrack so that you can shrink the viewing time to suit your schedule.

Technology, though, has done little to help us cope with the frenetic pace of our lives. As James Gleick, author of *Faster – The Acceleration of Just About Everything*, points out, labour-saving devices have been disappointing in the time saved. The dishwasher, for example, saves barely a minute in wash-up time, because people needlessly scour the dishes before placing them in the machine or they use more dishes. The kitchen whiz takes a lot longer to clean up than it does to work its magic.

If anything, technology is propelling us forwards at an even faster pace. Portable computers and cell phones make us instantly contactable – and the expectation is that we will respond with the same alacrity. And we do. We have become addicted to constant feedback and suffer withdrawal symptoms if deprived for even a short time. The first thing many passengers reach for as their plane hits the tarmac is their cell phone or PDA.

There is some evidence that our capacity to absorb more and more information and cope with the growing demands on our time is nearing its limit. Studies show that managing two or more mental tasks at once reduces the brain power available for each and takes longer than if you were to do them separately. University of Michigan psychology professor David Meyer has argued that multi-tasking '... increases errors, short circuits attention spans, induces air-traffic controller-like stress and elongates the time it takes to accomplish the most basic tasks by 50 per cent or more.'

Excessive multi-tasking can affect short-term memory and the prolonged adrenalin rush from it can damage cells that form new memory. In other words, we become more stupid.

Psychiatrist Edward M. Hallowell, an authority on Attention Deficit Disorder, used the term Attention Deficit Trait (ADT) to describe the 'distractibility, inner frenzy and impatience that results from trying to do too much at once'. In his book, *CrazyBusy*, he now refers to it as the '"F-State" because so many of the adjectives begin with the letter f: frantic, frenzied, forgetting, flummoxed, frustrated and fragmented, to name a few.'

Our reaction to overload, however, is not to cut back on our activities but to try to pack everything in more neatly, like a traveller with an overstuffed suitcase. We tell ourselves that if only we can make better use of our time we will cope. But as Hallowell says, 'Getting organized has become the modern form of dieting. Everyone wants to do it, few do it successfully, and even those who do it successfully usually revert to their former state.'

Before the 1980s, books on personal time management did not exist as a distinct publishing category. Now you'll find Amazon.com has a choice of 1356 titles, including *Time Management for Catholics*. (Time, indeed, seems to be a problem for Catholics; one study found that Catholics get more impatient than Protestants when they have to queue.)

'We've got ourselves so wound up into this state where our default option is always to go faster. We're afraid to slow down, because there's such a social taboo against it,' said Carl Honoré when I interviewed him about his bestseller, *In Praise of Slow*. A reformed speedaholic he may be, but he still talked like a man whose phone battery is about to die.

Honoré's book is a plea to put the brakes on; it documents

how a worldwide movement is challenging the cult of speed. Honoré blames turbocapitalism for our hurry sickness. 'These days, we exist to serve the economy, not the other way round.' To keep the wheels of the economy turning faster, we need to work longer hours and be persuaded to consume more and more products. However, the gadgets, the home-theatre system, the DVD recorder, the digital video camera, which were meant to compensate for the long hours we put in at work, only add to the clutter and time pressure of our lives, soaking up hours to set up, programme, maintain and accessorise. To misquote the *Bible*: for what doth it profit a man if he scores a top-of-the-range Bose sound system and does not have a decent CD collection or the time to listen?

There is no let-up in pace in our leisure time. As Robert Levine observes in his book, *A Geography of Time*, 'We live in a culture where it is not uncommon for people literally to run to relax, or to pay money for the privilege of pacing a treadmill.' We have been sold the idea that fast exercise is somehow virtuous and healthful. It's not a view shared by Drs Peter Axt and Michaela Axt-Gadermann. In *The Joy of Laziness* they say people, especially those in middle age and beyond, need to conserve energy not waste it in pointless strenuous exercise. Everyone, they argue, has a lifetime account of energy, a theory they support with reference to zoo animals. Some animals in captivity such as the lion and polar bear can more than double their lifespans, too big a difference to be accounted for by better medical care and the absence of predators. 'While wild animals cover many miles daily in search of food and consequently are under a great deal of stress, zoo animals lead a very restful and relaxed life.' If the couch potatoes of the animal kingdom live longer, why should humans be any different?

Research, however, does suggest that a lifetime of jogging, tennis and gym work will indeed extend your life – but only by about two years and you will have spent more than that length of time doing something you may not have enjoyed. 'Numerous studies have shown that a certain amount of movement protects us from circulatory disease and is good for our health. But athletic exercise isn't necessarily what we need,' say the two doctors.

Sports scientists are coming to appreciate that slower is often better. Studies have shown that we burn the most fat when our heart beats at 70 to 75 per cent of its maximum rate, the sort of effect achieved from power walking or light jogging. Walking also tones the whole body and its low impact reduces the risk of injury. And there are also countless examples of people who never took any exercise at all and survived well into their eighties and beyond.

Drs Peter Axt and Michaela Axt-Gadermann recommend eating less and even fasting to slow the body's metabolism and enjoy a longer, healthier life. And it's no coincidence, says Honoré, that the fastest nations are also the fattest. With no time to cook, we wolf down junk food. Since it takes 15 minutes for the brain to signal that you've eaten too much, the signal often comes too late, so it's easier to overeat without realising it.

'Slow food' is food that is savoured without guilt. In her book, *French Women Don't Get Fat*, Mireille Guiliano says that French women eat slowly and 'with all five senses'. 'French women take pleasure in staying thin by eating well, while American women see it as a conflict and obsess over it,' says Guiliano. British doctor Malcolm Kendrick theorises that the 400 per cent difference in coronary heart disease between Britain and France can be attributed to *how* the French eat rather than *what* they eat and drink, as is usually thought. Eating under stress, he argues, raises insulin levels and blood-sugar levels, 'which creates the metabolic state that triggers atherosclerotic plaque development'.

In a world that equates speed with power, efficiency and fun, we tend to be prejudiced against slow. People who are slow to process information are deemed to be less intelligent than those who grasp it immediately. As Hallowell, says 'In this fast world the slow processors can easily get dismissed, overlooked, or devalued. They are some of our wisest, most talented minds, and we do well to wait while they think, and stop and listen when they speak, even if they do so slowly.'

The slow movement is not a refuge for people who can't hack it in the fast lane. It's recognition that speed is sometimes inappropriate and counter-productive. In his book, *Hare Brain, Tortoise Mind – Why Intelligence Increases When You Think Less*, psychologist Guy Claxton argues that fast thinking, which is rational, analytical, linear and logical, can only take us so far. To come up with innovative and wise solutions to complex problems, we need to let things simmer in our unconscious. If you have no time to loaf or stare out the window, that's not going to happen.

'Research has shown that the tortoise mind can deal with problems that are more complicated than the hare brain can handle,' says Claxton. 'It takes a lot of "brain power" to break down situations into clear, well-articulated concepts and to manipulate them using conscious thought.' Because fewer ideas can be active in the brain at once, they tend to lack subtlety and shade. 'So, although hare-brain thinking feels more controlled, it may actually be working with a picture of a situation that is crude and even misguided . . . The more stressed people are, the more likely they are to fall back on the hare brain, and the more likely that approach is to fail.'

The paradox of slowness is that it often saves time. Honoré cites the case of German lawyer Erwin Heller, whose initial consultation with clients can last up to two hours. By getting to know the brief thoroughly and understanding his client's personality, circumstances, values, aims and fears, he has noticed that he needs to make fewer follow-up calls and doesn't have to backtrack because he has set off in the wrong direction. Doctors, too, are coming to appreciate that the 10-minute consultation with prescription pad in hand is failing patients, who are flocking to alternative medical practitioners who take the time to listen.

Honoré believes that speed in itself becomes a form of denial. 'The faster you go, the less time and tranquillity you have for thinking about the bigger questions: am I happy, is my family growing up in the right way, is my community functioning properly, are politicians making sensible decisions on my behalf? We're all so rushed that all this becomes just a blur. Speed becomes a form of running away from these questions because we sense below the surface that something's wrong, but we're scared to confront it.'

Our craving for speed can make us impatient over matters that don't lend themselves to quick solutions. How many couples split up and regret it later because they never allowed enough time to patch up their relationship? How much money is wasted on medical treatment for conditions that are self-limiting or are better treated over time through a change in lifestyle? We live in the age of the quick-fix. Self-help authors claim you can be wrinkle-free in three weeks, enjoy a satisfying sex life in 10 days, take charge of your emotions in 24 hours. Australian advertising executive Siimon Reynolds promises to change your life in your tea break with his book, *Become Happy in Eight Minutes.*

Not everyone feels the need to rush. Many countries in Africa, Asia, the Middle East and Latin America take a casual approach to time. 'Slowness is so ingrained in Mexican culture that people who abide by the clock invite insult,'writes Levine, who has devoted his career to studying time and the pace of life. In Brazil a three-hour wait is nothing. The Kayyle people of Algeria 'despise any semblance of haste in their social affairs, regarding it as a "lack of decorum combined with diabolical ambition"'.

Most of us, though, would be driven crazy by living in a world that lacked the stimulation of fast-paced modern life. As Levine says, there are benefits as well as downsides to being busy. 'People in faster environments are more prone to potentially deleterious stress as evidenced by higher rates of coronary heart disease; but they are also more likely to achieve a comfortable standard of living and, at least in part because of this, are more satisfied with their lives as a whole ... Working against the clock is not always stressful nor is the absence of time pressure inherently relaxing. Time pressure can be energizing and invigorating when served in the right dosage.'

The trouble is, we're seduced by the seemingly limitless possibilities on offer. We take on more than we can handle, gorge on the ever-present smorgasbord of pleasurable activities, and are dazzled by the distractions available at the touch of a button or the click of a mouse. Hallowell talks about 'screensucking, the way time can be frittered away watching TV, surfing the net, endlessly checking for emails, keeping up with the latest. In one of the many paradoxes of modern life the info addict loses his or her ability to make a difference in life by trying so hard to keep up with the differences other people are making.'

It's not going to get any easier. There will always be more TV channels to watch, more websites to visit, more opportunities to take advantage of. Unless we simplify and slow down, our lives are going to spin out of control. 'The best reason to *take your time* is that it is the only time you'll ever see,' writes Hallowell. 'You must take it or it will be taken from you.'

TEN

Choose to be Happy

The world would be a happier place if we all suffered a life-threatening illness. Invariably, people who survive such illnesses get a new perspective on life. They take less for granted. They are often happy just to be alive.

Happiness has a beneficial effect on our health. Our immune system fights disease more effectively than when we are depressed. When we are depressed, the number of disease-fighting cells declines. The link between hostility and heart disease is now well established. Moods matter. It's a truth that has been evident from ancient times. As the Book of Proverbs says, 'A cheerful heart is a good medicine, but a downcast spirit dries up the bones.' (That's not to say unhappiness is terminal: the number of grumpy old gits still collecting a pension in their eighties is proof of that.)

The trick is to learn to be happy. Some people have a head start. Studies of identical twins have found that 50 per cent of self-reported happiness can be marked down to genetic make-up. Extroverts are happier than introverts because as research shows they're more likely to get married, land good jobs and make new, close friends. Extroverts have been shown to have different brain activity than introverts.

More blood flows to their left front hemisphere, an area that helps generate positive emotions. They also appear to have a bigger right amygdala, the almond-shaped group of neurons that are involved in understanding emotional behaviour and feelings. Studies tracking the moods of extroverts and introverts across a normal week found that extroverts report their day's experience as happier and more pleasant.

If you're not naturally outgoing, though, there are still ways to boost happiness. Physical fitness helps. Aerobic exercise can boost positive emotions, possibly because of the release of endorphins and the fact that we tend to sleep better after exercise. Studies of mildly depressed people have shown that regular aerobic exercise can dramatically improve mental well-being.

As psychologist Dr Albert Ellis, originator of Rational Emotive Behaviour Therapy (REBT), says many people bring unhappiness – and ill health – on themselves through their own thoughts and attitudes. People have more choice over how they react to events than they give themselves credit for. For example, if a motorist swerves into your lane, forcing you to brake, you can blast the horn and fume about the 'offence' all the way to work, or you can shrug it off as the mistake of an inexperienced or inattentive driver.

'The human race,' argues Ellis, 'fools itself into believing (perhaps because of an innate propensity) that when you feel very upset then something must have caused you to feel it either in the present or in the past. However, almost always there is an intervening variable called your beliefs, your attitudes or your philosophy about the bad things.' There are no standard emotional reactions to life's events. What one person regards as a calamity, another may see as a minor setback. What separates humans from instinct-bound animals is the ability to consciously choose our reactions.

However, we have an innate bias towards negativity because it once bestowed evolutionary advantage. Worrying about predators or lack of food was more likely to ensure your survival than living a life cushioned by contentment. That negativity default can make life a misery if we fall into the habit of seeing or anticipating the negative side of everything. 'It will be a disaster if I don't get a promotion' is an irrational worry that is not going to affect the outcome. Likewise, statements such as 'I shouldn't have to put with this' or 'things never go right for me' are not based on objective reality. As therapist and REBT advocate Wayne Froggatt says in his book, *Choose to be Happy*, people need to question their beliefs: 'What grounds have I for believing that I, other people or things generally should, must or have to be the way I expect?'

Choosing our reactions rationally is a long way from the new-age belief in creating your own (happy) reality. 'We are not talking about so called "positive thinking",' writes Froggatt. 'Rational thinking is *realistic* thinking. It is concerned with facts – the real world – rather than subjective opinion or wishful thinking. Realistic thinking leads to realistic emotions. Negative feelings aren't always bad for you. Neither are all positive feelings beneficial. Feeling happy when someone you love has died, for example, may hinder your grieving properly. Or to be unconcerned in the face of real danger could put your survival at risk. Realistic thinking avoids exaggeration of both kinds, negative and positive.'

Nevertheless, optimists do tend to have better health and recover better from coronary bypass surgery and cancer. Harvard graduates, for example, who were the most pessimistic when interviewed in 1946, were least healthy when restudied in 1980. If you really want to be happy and healthy, get religion. There is a swag of studies supporting the link between religion and well-being. The two best indicators of well-being among older people are health and religion. Religious people cope better with crisis, are physically healthier and have greater self-esteem. The cost, however, may be too high for many. In *Civilization and its Discontents*, Freud argued that '... by forcibly fixing them in a state of psychical infantilism, and by drawing them into a mass delusion, religion succeeds in sparing many people an individual neurosis. But hardly anything more.'

One thing both religious leaders and social scientists agree upon is that money and possessions do not bring happiness. Despite rising incomes, shrinking family sizes, and doubled buying power in the US, for example, the number of Americans who reported that they 'were pretty well satisfied with your present financial situation' actually dropped from 42 per cent to 30 per cent. Affluence, as Seneca noted 2000 years ago, is a state of mind: 'No one can be poor that has enough, nor rich that covets more than he has.'

Over the past few years the study of happiness has become a growth industry, though it's doubtful whether we know any more about it than can be gleaned from philosophers like Seneca. In his book, *The Happiness Hypothesis*, social psychologist Jonathan Haidt set out to examine how ancient wisdom accords with what we now know from scientific research. For example, philosophers have long argued that external circumstances cannot have a long-term effect on our happiness. The modern study of hedonics suggests that we have a set point of happiness; our baseline happiness may fluctuate but after a short time it returns to what it was. Whether you win the lottery or become a paraplegic may not make that big a difference to your level of happiness, argues

Haidt. 'Of course, it's better to win the lottery than break your neck, but not as much as you'd think. Because whatever happens you're likely to adapt to it, but you don't realize up front that you will.'

Our hedonic set point, our incredible ability to quickly get used to new circumstances, is also why the pursuit of material things does not make us happier. No sooner have we acquired the plasma screen TV or the spa pool than it's taken for granted. To sustain that thrill of new possessions we need to acquire more and more; we're on what happiness researchers call the 'hedonic treadmill'.

But, as psychologist Martin Seligman points out in his book, *Authentic Happiness*, it's a futile exercise. Happiness, as philosophers have been telling us for millennia, comes from within. 'The belief,' says Seligman, 'that we can rely on shortcuts to happiness, joy, rapture, comfort and ecstasy, rather than be entitled to these feelings by the exercise of personal strengths and virtues, leads to legions of people who in the middle of great wealth are starving spiritually. Positive emotions alienated from the exercise of character leads to emptiness, to inauthenticity, to depression and, as we age, to the gnawing realisation that we are fidgeting until we die.' Seligman argues that knowing what our greatest strengths are and deploying them in the service of something we believe is larger than we are is what will make us happy over a lifetime.

In his influential book, *Flow: The Psychology of Optimal Experience*, Mihaly Csikszentmihalyi says it is only when we lose ourselves, and become totally absorbed in what we are doing, that we are truly happy. A happy life is a life with purpose, says Csikszentmihalyi. 'What is the meaning of life? turns out to be astonishingly simple. The meaning of life *is* meaning: whatever it is, whatever it comes from, a unified purpose is what gives meaning to life.'

Sometimes, though, it's the little things in life that make or break our happiness. Noise, over which we have no control, for example, can blight our lives (see 'Live the Quiet Life', page 95). Haidt says people who undergo plastic surgery, especially women who have breast enlargement or reduction, report high levels of satisfaction. Many have been painfully self-conscious their entire adult lives. 'Being freed from such a burden may lead to a lasting increase of self confidence and well being.'

In *The Consolations of Philosophy*, Alain De Botton's look at how philosophy can console, inspire and motivate us, he cites the case of the Renaissance essayist and thinker Michel de Montaigne. One of de Montaigne's great satisfactions was reflecting on life as he sat on the toilet. 'Of all the natural operations, this is the one during which I least willingly tolerate being disputed.' If asked to choose among the current glut of books on happiness, he might well have settled on the tome by Australian naturopath Peter Williams Edwards: *Happiness Is . . . A Regular Complete Bowel Motion.*

ELEVEN

Give Away Your Time

If you take a disabled person's car park, or badmouth a work colleague to get a promotion, are you being true to your deepest nature? In 1976, Richard Dawkins's hugely influential book, *The Selfish Gene*, claimed a biological basis for what philosophers and economists had been telling us for hundreds of years – that we are motivated only by self-interest, and altruism is merely disguised selfishness. 'A human society based simply on the gene's law of universal ruthless selfishness would be a very nasty society in which to live,' Dawkins wrote. 'But unfortunately, however much we may deplore something, it does not stop it being true.'

Recent research, though, suggests that even at gene level we may be capable of cooperation. Biologists investigating the green alga *Volvox carteri* have found that a gene called regA prevents single cells from growing and dividing in order to help other cells, which share some or all of its genes, to reproduce.

Research also suggests that our brains may be hard-wired to be cooperative and caring. A study led by Ernst Fehr, director of the Institute for Empirical Research in Economics at the University of Zurich, found that an area of the brain called the dorsolateral prefrontal cortex (DLPFC) helps people suppress selfish urges in unjust situations even if it's to their own disadvantage. The study involved 52 men in their twenties playing the 'Ultimatum Game', a standard experimental economics game in which two players have to share a sum of money. The first player decides how much money he wants to hand over, and the second whether he will accept the offer. If the second player rejects the share, neither gets anything. Many people playing the game will reject low offers because they are 'unfair'. In other words they act against their own self-interest to uphold the principle of fairness. In the Swiss experiment, the researchers 'switched off' the right DLPFC with a mild electric current. As a result, more than a third of the men accepted all of the unfair offers, while none of the control group (who did not receive a shock) accepted all of them.

While we may be programmed to play fair, other studies suggest that there are real physical and mental benefits from helping others. In fact, there may be no need to get off the couch to benefit from do-gooding. In the 1970s, psychologist David McClelland showed movies of Mother Teresa's work in Calcutta to his students to test if emotions have an effect on the immune system, as measured by changes in immunoglobulin A (S-IgA) in saliva, which protects us against colds and other respiratory diseases. To his surprise he found that the students all had elevated levels of S-IgA after viewing the film whether or not they admired Mother Teresa's work. A Nazi propaganda film, on the other hand, elicited no immune response. McClelland dubbed this the 'Mother Teresa Effect' (perhaps conveniently ignoring the fact that a film starring crusty misanthrope W. C. Fields also produced an immune response).

It's not known, though, whether a daily diet of Mother Teresa videos would maintain an improvement in immunity. It's possible you might suffer compassion fatigue by proxy. There's a lot of evidence, however, that actually doing things for other people has positive effects on well-being. In his 1991 book, *The Healing Power of Doing Good: The Health and Spiritual Benefits of Helping Others*, Allan Luks coined the phrase 'Helper's High' to describe the euphoria many volunteers experience after helping out. Luks had surveyed 3000 volunteers of all ages, more than 90 per cent of whom reported feeling elated, a rush that was followed by a period of emotional well-being after an act of altruism. The feel-good buzz returned for hours or even days whenever the volunteers remembered the helping act. More than 90 per cent of the volunteers reported increased feelings of self-worth, and 53 per cent said they were happier and more optimistic, and less prone to feeling depressed. The perceived health benefits increased with the frequency of volunteering. The pleasure, apparently, does not occur when merely donating money (though you'd think God would make an exception for Warren Buffett and his donation of $31 billion worth of shares).

Altruism may help us cope better with the vagaries of life. In his 1977 book, *Adaptation to Life*, based on a 30-year study of a group of Harvard graduates, psychiatrist George Vaillant noted that adopting an altruistic lifestyle seemed to have a critical role in mental health as the men reached their fifties.

The greatest benefits to be derived from volunteering may be in reconnecting with others. As Robert D. Putnam points out in *Bowling Alone*, his exhaustive study of the decline of social capital in the US, even animals who are kept in isolation develop more extensive atherosclerosis (hardening of the arteries) than less isolated animals. 'Over the last 20 years more than a dozen large studies of this sort in the United States, Scandinavia and Japan have shown that *people who are socially disconnected are between two and five times more likely to die from all causes, compared to matched individuals who have close ties with family, friends and the community.'*

That, of course, could be more of an argument for keeping close contact with family and friends rather than for volunteering. But Putnam goes on to cite many studies that show health benefits from volunteering and belonging to groups. 'The bottom line from this multitude of studies: As a rough rule of thumb, if you belong to no groups, but decide to join one, you cut your risk of dying over the next year *in half.* If you smoke and belong to no groups, it's a toss up statistically whether you should stop smoking or start joining. These findings are in some ways heartening: it's easier to join a group than to lose weight, exercise regularly, or quit smoking.' Putnam notes that while social connectedness has been declining, depression and even suicide have been increasing. 'Low levels of social support directly predict depression, even controlling for other risk factors, and high levels of social support lessen the severity of symptoms and speed recovery,' he says.

Paradoxically, while social capital declines and we become an increasingly self-obsessed society, more and more lip service is paid to altruism. Concern for the future of the planet or world poverty helps reposition our self-image as 'good people' rather than egocentric materialists. We rally to support good causes promoted by celebrities. There's a boom in 'voluntourism', combining a package holiday with voluntary work, usually in a deserving Third World country. As the website VolunTourism.org puts it, 'VolunTourism provides you with perspective and balance. You are able to utilize your "six" senses and interact with your destination in ways that had previously existed beyond your capacity of expectation. This is travel that unites your purpose and passion and ignites your enthusiasm in ways unimaginable.' In other words, it's all about you.

Volunteering of the authentic variety is surely about escaping from the prison of self, of not calculating what's to be gained, but helping because through that connection we become more human. The alternative is the myopic isolation of an ego that has no point of moral reference outside itself. We become like the Manhattan commuters so beautifully caught by John Updike in his novel, *Terrorist*: 'Scuttling, hurrying, intent in the milky morning sun upon some plan or scheme or hope they are hugging to themselves, their reason for living another day, each impaled live upon the pin of consciousness, fixed upon self-advancement and self-preservation. That and only that.'

TWELVE

Live the Quiet Life

It's well past midnight on a still summer's night. For the past hour you've been kept awake by the thump-thump of the teen-ager's heavy-metal music next door. It's barely audible but, no matter how much you try to ignore it, it remains irritatingly the focus of your attention. You get up and close the window. The room now feels hot and airless but the muffled beat is still there. You're becoming more and more frustrated and less and less inclined to sleep. An hour passes. God, how long is this noise going to go on?

Noise is one of the most pervasive pollutants. Unlike polluted air or water, we don't usually think about noise pollution as being potentially health damaging, but it can have profound effects on our physical and mental well-being. And its effect is all the more insidious because it is subjective and hard to fight. Noise does not have to be loud to affect us. Factors such as time and place, duration, and the source of the sound can make all the difference. The less control we have over it, the more likely it will do us harm.

It's easier to measure than to manage. Noise rises in decibels (dB). A whisper is 20 dB, normal conversation would register at about 65 dB, heavy traffic 70 dB, a jackhammer

100 dB, a jet engine 150 dB and so on. But the scale is logarithmic: every 10 dB increase will be perceived as twice as loud. And the closer you are, the louder the noise. A variable noise is more annoying than one that is constant. High-frequency noises can set our nerves on edge.

Noise has been the bane of people's lives for millennia. To ease traffic congestion in ancient Rome, chariots and wagons were allowed to move around the city only at night, creating a night-time hell for light sleepers as vehicles rattled through the streets, metal clanging on stone, and ungreased axles screeching. Our ancestors instinctively knew noise was harmful. The word 'noise' is derived from the same Latin root as the word 'nausea'.

Noise is everywhere. It's inseparable from modern life: the roar of traffic, the honk of horns, the squeal of air brakes, the rattle of trains, the thunder of planes overhead, the seesawing wail of sirens and car alarms, the clatter of cutlery and conversation in busy cafés, the omnipresent music of the shopping aisle, the jangle of cell phones and barking voices. There's no escape. Our homes, too, are hardly a refuge from noise. Dishwashers, extractor fans, washing machines, beeping fridges and microwave ovens compete with canned laughter from television sets, the din of electronic mayhem from game consoles or the blare of the radio or CD player. Outside, a motor mower drones in and out of earshot, there's raucous laughter, music, or the shrill of children from the patio next door. The fifteenth-century proverb 'Children should be seen and not heard' has something to recommend it. A childish scream can reach 90 dB, a banging toy as much as 110 dB. With the growing trend to treat gardens as outdoor rooms, the noise of neighbours' daily living is no longer shut out by walls. Barbecues, hot tubs and pools disturb the tranquillity of the suburban outdoors. Outdoor speakers concealed in plastic rocks pump secondhand noise through the shrubbery.

Acoustic stimulation has become a modern addiction. We are no longer the silent majority but the noisy majority. We can't seem to enjoy ourselves without a soundtrack. Living without noise seems as unnatural as watching TV with the mute on. We associate noise with power and effectiveness. In one study German housewives were invited to choose one of three vacuum cleaners. All were the same size and colour and had the same suction power. The only difference: each had a different degree of loudness. The women all chose the loudest vacuum cleaner because it seemed like the hardest-working and the most efficient. A similar experiment conducted with men using electric razors yielded the same results.

Over the past decades the quantity and volume of noise has increased dramatically. New technology allows us to amplify sound a great deal more without distorting it. Cinema sound levels, for example, have increased by 10–16 dB; in other words they have more than doubled in loudness since the 1950s, with some action movie scenes playing louder than a chainsaw at 130 dB. Car stereos are now able to pump out sound at levels high enough to blow out the windscreen. The world record for a car stereo system is 177 dB, about the same as a rocket taking off from a launch pad. State-of-the-art amplifiers used at pop concerts in the 1970s used to manage up to 300 W: now there are amplifiers that can handle 3000 W, a tenfold increase. A big concert might use up to 100 amplifiers.

Unfortunately, our ears are no match for modern technology. When noise reaches 80 db the muscles in the ear contract, reducing our sensitivity to the sound. This 'aural reflex' takes 10 milliseconds to occur, however; too late to prevent damage from the kind of noise that technology has made possible. As acoustic expert Rupert Taylor says in his book *Noise*, 'This type of impulse noise with a very short rise-time almost never occurs in nature, and is an exclusively man-made phenomenon. So nature has not really "slipped up" in allowing delay in the aural reflex, but has understandably not bargained for something which barely existed for millions of years.'

Our love affair with noise is polluting the planet. Silence is becoming an endangered experience. In 1984, acoustic ecologist Gordon Hempton was able to find 21 places in his home state of Washington that did not experience man-made noise for at least 15 minutes a day. Five years later he could find only three places. Even the oceans are noisy places. The giant container ships crisscrossing the world churn the water with their huge propellers causing millions of tiny bubbles, which then collapse with a thunderous hiss. Sonar surveys emit high-decibel sound waves that are suspected of harming whales, dolphins and porpoises.

Certainly, all the extra noise is harming us as a species. It's well known that cumulative long-term exposure to loud noise can damage our hearing, whether it's noise we have to endure at work or self-inflicted by maxing the volume on our iPods. If there's too much background noise we can't have a proper conversation, not because we can't hear what the other person is saying but because the noise is scrambling our brain activity. Recent research suggests that noise doesn't simply cover up sounds, it interferes with the brain's ability to process and interpret information about a sound even when it is received clearly.

But noise may affect not only our hearing but also our

general physical and mental health. Children and older people are the most vulnerable to the effects of noise. Studies show there is a correlation between high noise levels and low birth weight and possibly birth defects. Children who are exposed to constant noise can have difficulty learning. Noise in excess of 30 dB disturbs sleep. According to the WHO *Guidelines for Community Noise*, noise at that level will make it harder to get to sleep, cause us to wake more often, and reduce the number of restorative REM sleep periods. We will sleep less deeply and awake less refreshed. Noise during sleep can also cause our blood pressure to rise, increase our heart rate, change our breathing, and cause an increase in body movements during sleep.

A major German study published in the *European Heart Journal* found that general environmental noise of between 65 dB and 75 dB, such as that of traffic, increased the risk of heart attack by nearly 50 per cent for men and about 75 per cent for women. The lead researcher, Dr Stefan Willich, suggested noise was a mechanism that increased psychological stress and anger, which in turn increased the levels of adrenaline and noradrenaline, raising blood pressure. Evidence points to noise being a risk factor in lowering people's resistance to disease and infection. With raised stress levels, the body produces high levels of cortisol, which suppresses immune system functioning.

Noise has an adverse effect on our mental health. The literature suggests it can cause anxiety, emotional stress, nervous complaints, nausea, headaches, instability, argumentativeness, sexual impotency, changes in mood, and an increase in social conflicts, as well as general psychiatric disorders such as neurosis, psychosis and hysteria. Studies show that noise is linked to increased use of psychotropic drugs, and consumption of tranquillisers and sleeping pills. People subjected to noise complain of headaches, fatigue and stomach ulcers.

Noise can affect us even though we can't hear it. Infrasound at a frequency of 20 Hz is inaudible to most people but can have strange effects on the body. Research at NASA has found that infrasound causes people to hyperventilate and their eyeballs to vibrate. This can cause smearing of vision, which may result in hallucinations. You may see things out of the corner of your eye that don't exist. British scientists Vic Tandy and Tony Lawrence believe this phenomenon may explain why some people claim to see ghosts. In a paper, 'Ghosts in the Machine', Tandy recounted how he had seen a ghost in the laboratory where he was working but was eventually able to establish that his vision had been affected by the infrasound from a new extractor fan. 'When we switched it off, it was as if a huge weight was lifted,' he told the UK *Guardian*. Tandy believes infrasound may explain sick-building syndrome. A loose air-conditioning unit, for example, could produce low-frequency vibrations throughout the building. Exposure to excessive infrasound can cause a variety of mild to moderate disorders from repeated respiratory infections to gastrointestinal dysfunction and fatigue.

Infrasound can be generated by many different media, from wind and waterfalls to extractor fans and engines. Cathedral organ pipes are so long they can produce infrasound, creating an atmosphere during a service that churchgoers may believe is spiritual. Experiments using infrasound in a concert hall showed strange feelings, such as sorrow, coldness and anxiety could be instilled in an audience at will. One explanation for children getting sick in cars is that a car turning at speed causes the chassis to vibrate and create infrasound that causes nausea. Some scientists contend that excessive exposure to infrasound can cause vibro-acoustic disease, leading to a dangerous thickening of the heart walls and of the coronary blood vessels.

Though most people may never be exposed to noise long enough to cause permanent physical injury, there's little doubt that excessive noise does reduce the quality of our lives. Not being able to open a window at night or enjoy a peaceful moment in our garden makes life less pleasant and civilised. Noise isolates and makes us less sociable and helpful. In a series of experiments in the 1970s, researchers tested the helpfulness of pedestrians 'accidentally' dropping books on the pavement and seeing how many offered to pick them up. Eighty per cent of passers-by responded helpfully. However, when an 87 dB motor mower was switched on nearby, only 15 per cent of pedestrians offered assistance.

Noise may even be fattening; the stress can cause us to eat more. In one study conducted at Penn State University, study subjects ate more chocolate, cheese, popcorn and chips after being exposed to stressful noise. Even the noise of the cicadas, says one obesity expert, could prompt some stress-prone people to eat too much. It may pay to watch those decibels as well as those calories.

THIRTEEN

Take a Sonic Tonic

Six research teams in Europe and Canada are spending three years and millions of dollars to find out why music has such a profound effect on our emotional life, and how enjoying music and the emotions invoked by music are manifested in our brain functions. At last we'll know why millions of people buy Barry Manilow records!

To be fair, the Braintuning Project, as it's called, is far from frivolous. It should give us a deeper insight into why music has been found in every culture past and present. Nine-thousand-year-old flutes made from hollowed bird bones have been discovered in China, and what was believed to be a 45,000-year-old Neanderthal flute made of a hollowed bear bone was dug up in Slovenia in 1995. Music has been inseparable from civilisation since ancient times. The music of the lyre, it's said, kept Alexander the Great sane. The harp-playing of David calmed the agitated King Saul.

Like odours, music can sneak past our rational defences, conjuring up memories, evoking long-forgotten feelings and changing moods. Music with a slow tempo, low pitch, firm rhythm, and complex harmony is likely to provoke sad feelings. Faster music is more arousing and is likely to evoke happier feelings. Australian scientist Dr Emery Schubert has developed a mathematical formula to predict how a piece of music will affect the emotions. Loudness is the most powerful predictor of whether music will be arousing, followed by tempo. 'Our emotional response to music is highly complex – and has a lot to do with what we bring to the listening experience, such as memory, expectation and conditioning,' Dr Schubert says.

It's also becoming clear that music affects more than our emotions. Listening to Mozart is claimed to make children perform better academically. If only learning were that easy. On the other hand, there is some evidence that children who *study* music improve their general memory skills, which are correlated with non-musical abilities such as literacy, verbal memory, visio-spatial processing, mathematics and IQ. And there does seem to be something special about Mozart's music. In a study at the University of California, magnetic resonance imaging (MRI) was used to map regions of subjects' brains as they listened to Mozart, 1930s popular music and Beethoven's 'Für Elise'. As expected, all the music selections affected the auditory cortex, where the brain processes sound. Only the music of Mozart lit up the whole cortex.

In his book, *The Mozart Effect*, music therapist Don Campbell recommends using Mozart for a daily burst of what he calls 'sonic vitamin C'. It is believed that the high frequencies activate our brains and increase attentiveness. 'To create this effect, turn down the bass volume and, if you have a graphic equaliser, go for the mid-range on your sound system, and bring up the treble. Music with violins will help you obtain the most "nutritious" results.'

Our bodies have their own rhythms that respond to music. Classical music such as Pachelbel's *Canon* with its 60 beats a minute has a calming effect, slowing breathing and heart rate, and may help the lungs work more efficiently. Gregorian chant uses the rhythms of natural breathing and can relieve stress. Research published in the *Journal of Advanced Nursing* found that older people with sleep problems reported a 35 per cent improvement after they started listening to 45 minutes of soft music before bedtime. Speed up the music and your body becomes energised. Playing music at about 140 beats a minute while walking, for example, will help you maintain a brisk pace and improve aerobic fitness.

Music can lower your blood pressure, at least temporarily. Studies have found that in intensive care units where music is playing, heart-bypass surgery patients require lower doses of drugs to control their often erratic blood pressure. More and more hospitals are discovering the therapeutic benefits of music. The Exempla Good Samaritan Medical Center in Colorado, for example, is equipped with a sound system with 16 different zones. Bird sounds are piped into faux rocks by the hospital's entrance to evoke a calming, optimistic feeling in visitors. In the surgery waiting rooms, they play a selection of baroque concerts; in radiology, it's classical strings; and the emergency department has relaxing ambient music. When a baby is born in the hospital, the whole system switches for 10 seconds to Brahms's 'Lullaby'.

Music is now routine in many operating theatres. Studies suggest music makes surgeons calmer, more accurate and speedier, can help reduce the amount of sedation needed for some patients, and lower blood pressure in others. According to a *New York Times* report: 'Loud rock 'n' roll is good for routine operations ... Mozart for trickier ones. There is even a genre called "closing music": raucous sounds to suture by.' Patients can also request music to be played during an operation. When US President Bill Clinton tore a tendon in 1997 and chose to undergo the operation without a general anaesthetic, he asked for the operating room to be filled with country and western music. Proof, perhaps, that healing sounds are in the ear of the beholder.

Even the unborn are moved by music. In his 1982 book, *The Secret Life of the Unborn Child*, Dr Thomas Verny writes: 'In an arresting series of new studies audiobiologist Michele Clements has shown that the unborn child has distinct musical likes and dislikes and discriminating ones at that. Vivaldi is one of the unborn child's favorite composers; Mozart is another. Whenever one of their soaring compositions was put on, reports Dr Clements, fetal heart rates invariably steadied and kicking declined. The music of Brahms and Beethoven and all kinds of rock, on the other hand, drove most fetuses to distraction. They kicked violently when records of these composers were played to their pregnant mothers.' So much for Brahms's 'Lullaby'.

Music has been used in neonatal wards to help premature babies thrive. Kosice-Saca Hospital in Slovakia is famous for its infant music therapy. Newborns are tuned into Mozart via headphones, which staff say stabilises breathing, relieves pain and stress, and helps them to gain weight.

But perhaps the greatest benefit of music therapy has been for people with conditions such as Alzheimer's and Parkinson's disease. Neurologist and author Oliver Sacks is a firm believer in the power of music after experiencing it for himself. In 1982 he had a bad fall from a mountain in Norway that damaged the muscles and nerves in one leg. He lost not only the use of the leg, but also any feeling that the 'bizarre appendage' actually belonged to him. It was only when Mendelssohn's 'Violin Concerto' played in his mind that he was able to not only regain the art of walking but also an awareness of the damaged limb as part of him. As he wrote in his book, *A Leg to Stand On*, hearing the inner music changed everything. 'And as suddenly, without thinking, without intending whatever, I found myself walking easily *with* the music ... and in that very moment my "motor" music, my kinetic melody, my walking came back – in the self-same moment, *the leg came back.*'

Music, says Sacks, has the same effect on the neurologically impaired, at least for the time that it lasts. 'For reasons we do not yet understand, musical abilities often are among the last to be lost, even in cases of widespread brain damage. Thus someone who is disabled by a stroke or by Alzheimer's or another form of dementia may still be able to respond to music in ways that can seem almost miraculous.'

Music therapy is not confined to Western culture. The Chinese have adapted traditional Chinese music and released a number of music therapy albums, with titles such as *Constipation, Liver Heart and Lungs* and *Obesity*. In India, traditional *raga* melodies have been used in therapy. Doctors, neurologists and psychiatrists at the Raga Research Centre in Madras have found that certain *ragas* are beneficial in treating hypertension and mental illness.

For most of us, though, the effect of music on our health is likely to be small but still very worthwhile – an aid to relaxation, a mood changer, a lasting pleasure. Music has been touted as a useful pain reliever, but the effect appears to be quite small. A Cochrane Review of Evidence-based Healthcare analysed 51 clinical studies and found that patients reported, on a scale of 0–10, only an average drop of 0.5 in the intensity of their pain as a result of listening to music.

Still, there are many true believers who argue otherwise.

Don Campbell claims the human voice can also be useful in healing: 'All forms of vocalisation, including singing, chanting, yodelling, humming, reciting prose or poetry or simply talking can be therapeutic.' Yodelling when you have a headache may attract unwanted attention, but a quiet hum can apparently be effective if you find the tone that is unique to you. Combined with two aspirin it will do wonders for your headache.

FOURTEEN

Get Down to Earth

The garden is bursting into life. The ornamental cherry tree is covered in pink blossom and there are buds on the bare branches of the birch. The rhododendron planted to mark the birth of our first child (the custom lapsed before the arrival of the other two) is in full bloom. Leaving for work when it's barely light and returning after dark, I'm hardly aware of the changes. In any case I'm not much of a gardener; I wouldn't know my azalea from my euphorbia. The thought of gardening conjures up chores of weeding, mowing, trimming. Time begrudged, time that could more profitably be spent reading, writing or cleaning up my hard drive. Yet even I have been known to experience the odd moment of affinity with nature, of wonder at the endless cycle of decay and renewal – and that's just from contemplating the stuff at the back of the fridge.

Gardening is health-giving. It won't cure cancer or prevent diabetes, but it can bring a powerful sense of well-being. Gardening has become a recognised therapy beneficial to mental patients. In the early 1800s, a Scottish physician by the name of Dr Gregory became famous for curing insanity by putting his patients to work on a farm. In the past, poor people often worked in gardens to pay for their hospitalisation, and doctors noticed that these patients recovered more quickly and to a better health standard than other patients. Dr Benjamin Rush, the famous American physician of his day, wrote in 1812: 'It has been remarked that maniacs of the male sex in all hospitals who assist in cutting wood, making fires and digging in the garden ... often recover while persons whose rank exempts them from performing such services, languish away their lives within the walls of the hospital.' (Washing, ironing and scrubbing was deemed good therapy for maniacs of the female sex.)

Wounded soldiers from World Wars I and II were often encouraged to work in gardens to improve both the functioning of their injured limbs and mental condition. Recent research has shown that hospital patients recover more quickly from surgery when they have a view of grass and trees. Prisoners whose cells overlook green spaces have fewer bouts of sickness. Even videos of pastoral scenes were shown in one study to reduce anxiety, pulse rate, muscle tension and blood pressure in stressed people. In one Swedish study, three groups of post-operative heart patients were either given a landscape painting or an abstract painting to look at, while a control group had no painting to look at. The patients who looked at the landscape experienced lower anxiety, needed less pain relief, and spent a day less in hospital than the other groups. Those who looked at the abstract painting actually felt sicker, more anxious, and initially needed more painkillers than the control group.

If mere images of nature are healing, the real thing surely has added benefits. 'Recent research in environmental psychology,' reported the *British Medical Journal*, 'is now giving encouragement to the call for the revival of the old tradition of providing gardens for hospital patients.' Horticultural therapy is now widely used with patients to alleviate depression and improve motor skills. A three-year study completed in 2005 by Britain's Loughborough University evaluated the health and well-being benefits of gardening for disabled and disadvantaged adults. The study found that gardening provided a restorative environment that increased self-confidence and self-esteem and made them feel better both physically and psychologically.

In his book, *The Therapeutic Garden*, Donald Norfolk argues that gardening is beneficial not only for the sick and disabled, but also for all of us. Our resistance to disease, says Norfolk, may be enhanced by regular association with the soil. Such contact with the countless bacteria in the earth is prophylactic, because it triggers a defensive immune reaction that helps raise our resistance to infection, and reduces our resistance to allergies and auto-immune disease. An afternoon of gardening will burn up about 1000 calories and improve physical fitness, and cardiovascular and muscle strength. Gardening is meditation and stress-relief in motion. Environmental psychologist Professor Clare Cooper Marcus has said: 'When you are looking intensely at something or you bend down to smell something, you bypass the [analytical] function of the mind.'

A 2001 University of Illinois study showed that time spent in green, natural surroundings helped children with attention deficit disorder to concentrate and complete tasks. It may also benefit increasingly distracted adults. The researchers noted: 'The ability to deliberately pay attention ... draws on voluntary attention. Like a mental muscle, voluntary attention becomes fatigued with exertion. To refresh and renew this mental muscle, the use of involuntary attention is effective. Involuntary attention is effortless ... Simply noticing the sights, sounds and scents of the environment exemplifies it. Studies of adults have shown that time spent in nature uses involuntary attention especially effectively. Voluntary attention rests, and the ability to concentrate is renewed.'

The American playwright Arthur Miller used gardening as a form of moral and occupational therapy. 'Whenever life seems pointless and difficult to grasp, you can always get out in the garden and get something *done*. Also, your paternal and maternal instincts come into play, because helpless living things are depending on you, require training and encouragement and protection from enemies.'

As the father of teenagers, I get enough of 'helpless living things'. What's more appealing is the solitude of the garden, for what self-respecting teenager would willingly venture out of doors before dark? As Norfolk points out, most people in Western countries spend 85 to 95 per cent of time indoors; we are becoming a new species – *homo encapsularis*. 'When we are working indoors, the optimum temperature for comfort is several degrees higher than for peak brain function. A cold shower can increase metabolism by 80 per cent, bringing a fresh flow of blood to the brain. Exposure to the wind has a similar effect: a gentle breeze of just 5 mph cools the body by a third or more, which empties the reservoirs of blood within the skin and increases the circulation to the heart, brain and other vital organs. This can provide a vigorous boost to mental activity, which is why we often think better, and are more creative, when we are exposed to the fresh air.'

You can have your garden and eat it too. Geophagy, the fondness for eating dirt, is often considered aberrant behaviour, but the practice is common across many cultures.

Pregnant women are the most likely to consume clay, and scientists say it may be beneficial because it can contain high levels of calcium, iron, copper and magnesium, essential minerals for the human diet, especially during pregnancy. Eating clay (subsoil, not bacteria-ridden topsoil) can also alleviate nausea and morning sickness, and build up the immune system. Silicate minerals from clay are the active ingredients in diarrhoea medication. Clay has a detoxifying effect, removing alkaloids and tannic acids from foods and making them more palatable, which may be why clay vessels were often traditionally used for cooking.

It's a pity we can't eat grass; it might give us more incentive to cut it. The joys of gardening have been somewhat reduced by the tyranny of lawn care. In 1919, an American army colonel called Edwin George invented the gasoline-powered lawn mower. As a result of his thoughtlessness, peaceful weekends all over the world have been destroyed by the whine of motor mowers, the smell of two-stroke, the oaths and curses when the ridiculous machines splutter to a halt. The cult of the perfect lawn has bred an intolerance, not only of other plants, but of people. There are children growing up in the more select suburbs who have never seen a dandelion puffball, who have come to associate weeds and long grass with people from lower socio-economic groups. In their minds, the great unwashed go hand in hand with the great unweeded. Nothing angers the parents of these children more than neighbours who flout convention by not mowing their lawns. A bit of domestic violence can be ignored by turning up the TV a little louder, but a neglected weed-ridden lawn next door is seen as an affront and a threat to civilisation, bringing down property values.

Needless to say, people who buy into such conformist

attitudes and beliefs will never enjoy the therapeutic benefits of gardening. As Norfolk says, garden time should be spent hunkering down to smell the flowers, striking a balance between exertion and restful contemplation. 'The wilder the garden the better it will serve its therapeutic purpose. The less you curb, control and cosset it, the more it will flourish.'

As we grow older, the world seems to make less and less sense, and be less amenable to reasoned argument. We watch impassioned debates on TV about the latest Middle East conflict or global warming and sigh. Like Voltaire's Candide, we are inclined to say, 'All that is very well, now let's cultivate our garden.'

FIFTEEN

Read for Your Life

As a teenager I was almost driven to suicide by literature. I was depressed by the bleak poetry of T. S. Eliot, morally jaundiced by Sartre's *Nausea*, and turned cynical by Salinger's *A Catcher in the Rye*. I remember being stirred when one of my favourite fictional characters, Jack London's Martin Eden, decides in the last pages of the novel to kill himself. 'When life became an aching weariness, death was ready to soothe away to everlasting sleep. But what was he waiting for? It was time to go.' When you're 17, trapped in a hick town in Northern Ireland and your girlfriend has gone off with some stupid oaf in a leather jacket, it's hard not to take such words to heart.

'Good' literature can be dangerous and unhealthy stuff. When Goethe published *The Sorrows of Young Werther* in 1774 it's said to have inspired scores of copycat suicides across Europe that continued not for a year but for decades. If socio-paths were more literate, Anthony Burgess's *A Clockwork Orange*, published in 1962, might have provoked a series of copycat violent crimes. In the event, it was Stanley Kubrick's 1971 film adaptation that was blamed for initiating crimes, including the rape of a Dutch girl by men harmonising 'Singing in the Rain'. On the whole, though, literature is sustaining and life-affirming, a cure for the psychic pain, depression and emptiness that can engulf us all.

Poetry therapy and bibliotherapy are now recognised methods of healing sick minds and helping people gain perspective or endure mental and physical trauma. Poetry is sometimes regarded as other-worldly, too whimsical to have any real use. 'The truth is that poetry is, in fact, one of the most effective "grounding" mechanisms that exists,' writes American psychiatrist Jack Leedy, author of the definitive works on the subject, *Poetry Therapy* and *Poetry the Healer*. (The word therapy comes from the Greek word *therapeia*, meaning to nurse or cure through dance, song, poem and drama.)

For someone who feels utterly alone with their problems, poetry can be a revelation. A poet, perhaps centuries ago, had felt that same despair, anger or sorrow and described it precisely. As one poetry therapist put it, 'poetry humanizes because it links the individual by its distilled experience, its rhythms, its words to another in a way which no other form of communication can. Poetry also helps to ease the aloneness which we all share in common.' In *Once In A House on Fire*, Andrea Ashworth's searing memoir of growing up in a violent and abusive family in the slums of Manchester, she recalls how poetry kept her sane and taught her to see value in her world. 'I worshipped Philip Larkin, who got stuck into the dullest corners of life and picked up ordinary, everyday stuff to smack you with art.'

Poetry often helps depressed people to open up: when they are talking about the poem, their own emotions well up. Poetry doesn't have to rhyme, but it must have rhythm. Verses match the poet's body rhythms, and it's said that the poets we tend to like best are those whose body rhythms match our own. A few books of poems should be up there, with the indigestion tablets, the aspirin and calamine lotion in our medicine cupboard. 'A well-chosen anthology,' said the poet Robert Graves, 'is a complete dispensary of medicine for the most common mental disorders and may be used as much for the prevention as cure.'

In Britain, a charity called Poems in the Waiting Room distributes pamphlets of poetry to more than 3000 GPs' waiting rooms, including works by Dylan Thomas, W. B. Yeats, Wordsworth, Sir John Betjeman, Ted Hughes, Spike Milligan and Roger McGough.

Some UK doctors are sending their patients to the library instead of the pharmacy. Prescribing self-help books instead of antidepressants has been a key recommendation of the British National Institute for Clinical Excellence, which has become concerned at the over-prescribing of drugs for mild and moderate depression.

Getting patients to read self-help literature fits neatly into our age of makeover and DIY. Reframe your mental outlook, jettison that emotional baggage, gain a new perspective, feel good about your life. It may sound like wishful thinking, but there is some evidence that self-help books do work for mild or moderate conditions. 'Recent US reviews,' writes Professor David Richards in the *Journal of Mental Health*, 'suggest that "self treatment" through bibliotherapy in depression and anxiety achieve effects roughly equivalent to the average achieved in studies of psychotherapy.'

Unfortunately, many of the books that set out directly to solve the reader's problems are written primarily to increase the author's bank balance. As Wendy Kaminer, author of *I'm Dysfunctional, You're Dysfunctional*, observed, the only difference between a self-help reader and a self-help writer may be 'that the writer can write well enough to get a book deal'.

'The messages [of self-help books] are so vague and so general that there's really no way to apply it to your life. It's just a lot of feelgood blather that doesn't really mean anything in the end,' says Steve Salerno, author of *SHAM*, a critique of the self-help movement.

In fact, some self-help books intended as parodies of the genre contain more sensible advice than those offered in po-faced seriousness. Who could argue with Rich Hall when he advises in his *Self Help for the Bleak*: 'When someone says, "It's better to have loved and lost than never to have loved at all", keep in mind you're talking to a loser. Try to find someone who's never loved at all and get their side of the story.' Even if a self-help book does offer sound advice, you have to feel comfortable with it. Positive affirmations may work for some people, but no matter how miraculous the results I think I'd find it hard to repeat to myself every morning in the shaving mirror: 'I have a nice smile. I'm a fun brother to be around. I'm smart. My game is tight.'

Self-help books can feed a self-obsession that in the long run is guaranteed to make you unhappy. The antidote to that is reading good fiction, which broadens our perspective, simulates situations that provide us with models of behaviour, and allows us to enter mentally into the experience of other people. One study found that readers of fiction had a greater empathy for people and greater social awareness than readers of non-fiction. Good fiction can ease our dis-ease. 'A book,' wrote Kafka, 'should serve as an axe for the frozen sea within us.'

Fiction can help us understand the tangle of emotions, motivations and self-justifications we experience in a way that the simplistic scenarios in self-help books never can. Tolstoy's great novel, *Anna Karenina*, for example, speaks to many women going through a marital crisis. John Updike's Rabbit Angstrom novels present an everyman at once repellent and familiar, an ordinary fallible man against whom we can measure our own lives. We identify with these people because they are like us – people who will never acquire '7 Highly Effective Habits' or conquer '4 Self-Defeating Behaviours'.

Perhaps literature is so therapeutic because many writers have personally struggled with their demons and experienced the pain of loss or failure. Male writers have been shown to have high rates of mood disorders and alcoholism. In the US, a University of Kentucky Medical Center researcher sampled 59 female writers attending a women writers' conference. The psychiatric problems of the women writers were then compared with non-writers of similar background. The survey showed that 59 per cent of the writers had suffered from depression compared with only 14 per cent of the non-writers. Other comparisons were equally dramatic: mania 19 per cent/3 per cent; panic attacks 22/5; eating disorders 12/2; drug abuse 17/5; and childhood sexual abuse 39/12. 'It is quite possible,' Noam Chomsky has said, 'that we will always learn more about human life and personality from novels than from scientific psychology.' (Perhaps, though, it needs to be repackaged for our therapeutic age. Would Dostoevsky's *Notes from the Underground* fly off the shelves with a new title such as *Chicken Soup for the Alienated Soul*?)

Good fiction lends us perspective, enriches our understanding, and sustains us through communion with other human beings. It can be a comfort and a refuge, transporting us to a different world. I can still recall the sense of loss I felt as an unhappy teenager at boarding school as I closed *David Copperfield* for the last time. As Victor Nell says in *Lost in a Book: The Psychology of Reading for Pleasure*, 'Reading for pleasure is an extraordinary activity. The black squiggles on the white page are as still as the grave, colourless as the moonlit desert; but they give the skilled reader a pleasure as acute as the touch of a loved body, as rousing, colourful and transfiguring as anything out there in the real world.'

Family

A family is a unit composed
not only of children
but of men, women, an
occasional animal, and
the common cold.

OGDEN NASH
US HUMORIST AND POET (1902–1971)

SIXTEEN

Screen Your Genes

It ain't fair. You can eat all the right things, exercise regularly, avoid stress, and have regular medical check-ups – and still contract some debilitating, life-threatening disease. Who's to blame? Your family. No matter what you do, you cannot escape your genetic inheritance. There are more than 3000 genetic disorders; many very rare, some very common. Major diseases such as heart disease, cancer and diabetes show a tendency to run in families. If you have a relative who had a heart attack before reaching 65, your risk of having one before that age is seven times higher than normal. Some cancers are known to be directly inherited, for example, retinoblastoma of the eye, a rare cancer that develops in children.

All of us have faulty genes, but most disorders are more likely to occur only when both parents transmit the same faulty gene. Genetic disorders can be passed down the generations like perverse family heirlooms. In her book *How Healthy Is Your Family Tree?*, Carol Krause tells the story of a woman who gave birth to a dwarf. Told that it was genetic, the woman was emphatic that dwarfism had not occurred in either her or her husband's family. She set out to prove the genetic specialist wrong by tracing her family tree. 'Because her family had some minor royalty back in England she was able to trace them back to the 18th century. That's when she found him. A great-great-great-great-great-grandfather actually served as a court jester at an important royal palace. Although he was a nobleman himself, he was of dwarfish stature.'

Who knows what rogue genes lie dormant in our genetic cupboard? Take the case of malignant hyperthermia or MH, a hereditary condition in which certain anaesthetics can make the patient's temperature soar, causing massive damage to heart, liver and other organs. MH can be the reason that seemingly healthy children or adults die under routine anaesthesia. Some genetic diseases, such as Huntington's disease, don't show up until middle age. Huntington's is a steady degeneration of the brain cells that causes uncontrollable movements, intellectual impairment and, in some cases, emotional disturbance. It's possible to have a highly accurate test for Huntington's, but many people prefer not to know they carry the defective gene.

You can buy genetic testing kits on the Internet that claim to show if you have 'risky' genes and whether you are likely to get cancer, coronary artery disease, or other life-threatening disorders. All that's required is to post off a swab of cheek cells or in some cases a blood sample. Two weeks later you get the results along with advice on how to live a healthier life. A genetic test claiming to 'help identify your body's nutritional needs' is also sold through Body Shop stores in the UK.

These 'health horoscopes' have been widely condemned by health authorities who say that complex diseases cannot be predicted with simple tests. As one British doctor put it, 'Just looking at genes can't really tell you that much about your risk of certain diseases because the prediction hasn't got lifetime exposure to environmental risk factors built into it'. Even if the tests show that you're predisposed to certain diseases, it doesn't mean you will get them. People with a variation in the ApoE gene associated with the development of Alzheimer's, for example, don't always develop the disease, and people who don't have this mutation may still get it.

Despite the fact some are often little more than horoscopes, genetic tests are used in the US for screening prospective employees. According to one survey, some employers conduct genetic testing to check for such diseases as sickle-cell anaemia, Huntington's, and breast and colon cancer. Many also collect family medical history, an important source of genetic information. One company required employees who developed carpel tunnel syndrome to undergo genetic testing, presumably to argue that the injuries of 'predisposed' employees were not sufficiently work-related to be eligible for compensation.

There's a risk that people will find themselves dis-criminated against because of their genes, not only by employers, but also by insurance companies. In Britain, health authorities feared that some people who had a strong family history of certain diseases were not having tests because they feared the results would be used to deny them insurance. (In the US some people have genetic testing done under false names.) The British insurance industry has agreed to an extended moratorium on using genetic tests for insurance assessment until 2011. The rationale for the moratorium is that genetic testing is a relatively new science and the ethical and social implications have yet to be debated. It has also been argued that since genetic testing is available for only about 200 of the estimated 6,000 single gene disorders, it is unfair to single out people affected by the few diseases for which we can now test. A British government white paper on genetics estimates that 'six out of 10 people are likely to develop a disease that is at least partially genetically determined by age 60'. Already there is talk of a 'genetic superclass' of the well and insurable and a 'genetic underclass' of the unwell and uninsurable.

The fact that certain diseases run in the family, though, does not have to be a cause of despair and hopelessness or a reason not to adopt a healthy lifestyle. Knowing that breast cancer, diabetes or glaucoma is part of the family history can be invaluable in alerting us to watch for early warning signs. It's also possible to avoid diseases that we may be genetically disposed towards by changing our lifestyles. For instance, one study showed that men whose mothers died of a stroke face three times the usual risk of dying from the disease. My mother died from a stroke, but I hope to avoid that fate by keeping my blood pressure down through weight control and regular exercise. Being a non-smoker also lessens the risk.

The more you know about your family medical history, the fewer surprises may be in store. Forget asking Great Aunt Jane about her school days; quiz her instead about seizures, dislocated hips at birth, allergies, gallbladder problems, unusual reproductive organs, varicose veins, webbing of toes or fingers, alcoholism, cysts/ lumps/growths/tumours and the like. When viewed genetically, family members can be seen in a new light. Grandpa Ron, a bit of a character, becomes a left-handed diabetic with a weight problem and protruding ears.

In the US, the Surgeon General has dubbed Thanksgiving Day as National Family History Day to encourage Americans to use their family gatherings as a time to collect important family history. Which may make for some unusual dinner-table conversation. 'Didn't you once have a benign urethral lesion, Dad?'

The family photo album may also yield clues to possible inherited diseases. As one family sleuth put it, 'Short family members with smallish heads, think celiac disease ... family members who are overweight, with sallow complexions and the loss of their outer third eyebrow, think under-active thyroid especially if they are deaf or hoarse ... average height, unusually thin, think milk and grain allergies.' An American study found that people with small head size and the gene variant apolipoprotein E e4 (ApoE e4) are 14 times more likely to develop Alzheimer's disease than people without that combination.

Fossicking in the family closet can reveal not only medical weak points but also shed light on behaviour and personality. The genes you inherit from your parents play a major role in shaping your personality. The famous Minnesota Twins study, which tested hundreds of sets of twins, including 44 sets of identical twins, found compelling evidence that it is genes rather than environment that is the most important factor in how we and our children turn out. Based on the findings about twins, researchers were able to estimate how much genes influenced behaviour in the general population.

Traits such as extroversion, creativity, conformity, orderliness and paranoia owe as much to nature as to nurture. If you're onto your third marriage, it may not be entirely your fault or your previous partners'. To get a better picture of who is at fault, you may need to draw up a genogram, a family tree that displays not only medical history but also relationship patterns recurring across generations. Genograms can include everything: physical, mental and emotional issues, extramarital relationships, job losses, feuds, psychological disorders such as gambling, cross-dressing and so on. To misquote Tolstoy: Every family is unhappy, ill and dysfunctional in its own way.

SEVENTEEN

Survive the Family

Mum's new boyfriend Barry, a used-car salesman with aspira-
tions, wants to invest her savings in a Nigerian get-rich-quick
scheme. At the end of the table, Uncle Toby, the corners of his
mouth flecked with beer foam, is regaling his young nephews
with tales of his exploits as a white supremacist party activist.
On the couch, 14-year-old Kylie in halter top and mini-skirt is
shamelessly turning on Grandpa, gyrating like a lap dancer
on his knee to the beat of her iPod.

Families should carry a health warning: prolonged
exposure will dangerously elevate your blood pressure,
induce stress-related illnesses and impair your mental
health or psychologically scar you for life. It's not just
having to relate to people with whom we no longer have
a lot in common; families also have a way of unearthing
old hurts and anxieties that we thought we had long put
behind us. 'Families are similar to a theatrical drama. Like
fictional characters, we are each assigned a scripted role,
tightly directed in its performance, clothed in psychological
costumes and required to sing and dance to our family tune.
This is proven whenever there is a family gathering, at
Christmas, for example,' observes British psychiatrist Oliver

James in his book, *They F*** You Up: How to Survive Family Life*.

James's title is from Philip Larkin's famous line, 'They fuck you up, your mum and dad.' Though some people prefer the sunnier parody, 'they tuck you up, your mum and dad', James is convinced that Larkin got it exactly right. Forget genetics, it's family life that makes us what we are, he argues. 'Parental care is critical, especially during the first six years. The patterns of brain electro-chemistry created then are brought to bear in choosing friends, lovers and professions, and in constantly recreating the patterns of the past. The earlier the pattern was established, the harder it is to change.' People such as Woody Allen, Elton John, Ruby Wax and Prince Charles, notes James, didn't get to be what they are today by having reasonable or loving parents.

Outward appearances can be deceptive. Parents who bask in the success of their high-achieving children may not realise that they have turned them into insecure, unhappy wrecks who suffer from Dominant Goal Depression, which can only be alleviated by the arid pursuit of more 'success'. 'An in-depth British study,' writes James, 'compared academically high-flying, middle-class girls with working-class ones from the age of four. All the middle-class girls were considerably more anxious and stressed by the age of nineteen. Despite mostly having done very well, they still felt they had not achieved enough.'

But if parental high expectations have their hazards, the unfavoured child fares even worse. 'At least one in 10 children report that one of their parents "really seemed to dislike me or have it in for me",' writes James. A major hurdle to many children's life chances is the inequality in society: the children of the well-off often have an unassailable lead for life. However, in his book, *The Pecking Order*, US sociologist Dalton Conley argues that inequality begins at home. America, he says, is the most unequal developed country in the world. 'Given the level of disparities, it becomes all the more striking that more of the inequality in American society is attributable to differences within families – i.e. between siblings.'

Though Conley's analysis is focused on America, his findings are relevant to any developed country. We often regard the family as the best ally in realising a child's potential, but it often does not work for all the siblings. Instead of helping children get an equal chance in life, the family can increase disparity of opportunity. The gifted or talented child gets the lion's share of family resources. The younger children in large families receive less attention and affection from harried and tired parents. Tired parents are also less likely to put a stop to sibling abuse, which has been called the most accepted and ignored form of family violence. Children may not be born like piglets with 'needle teeth' to attack their litter-mates, but they can still make life a misery for their weaker and smaller siblings. Children are labelled as clever or awkward or scatter-brain, tags that may determine their self-image and self-confidence across a lifetime. Brothers marry and move away, leaving their sister to shoulder alone the burden of caring for sick or ageing parents.

If family does not always improve the well-being of all children, parents too may also be impaired by the experience. A study of 13,000 US parents published in the *Journal of Health and Social Behaviour* found that parents are more likely to be depressed than those who have no children. Even parents whose children have moved out of the family home, the empty nesters, are more likely to be depressed. The least depressed were parents with young children, perhaps because they didn't know what lay ahead.

It's hardly surprising that parenting can be damaging to your health. Parents receive lots of blame but little credit. In *The Nurture Assumption*, for example, psychologist Judith Harris claims that how children turn out depends a lot more on genetics and peer influence than on parenting. In other words, parental sacrifices of time and money make little difference and, as every parent of teenagers knows, are little appreciated by the recipients. It also quickly becomes clear to parents that when society leaders talk about the importance of parenting and family values they are mouthing platitudes. Spending more time with the family is apparently what politicians and other worthies yearn to do, but it only becomes a priority when their careers are on the skids and there's nothing else on offer. Likewise, employers pay lip service to the importance of family, but promotion goes to those who are prepared to always put the job ahead of their personal life, who are always first in the office and last to leave. Workplaces make few concessions to the needs of parents who have to juggle their children's timetables with their own, and the days are long gone when most families could manage on a single income.

What little family time remains after work is crowded out with domestic chores such as cooking and cleaning. Ironically, in the US, where family values have long been a favourite theme of politicians, family members have the least time for each other. 'In the most recent study of American family time, it was discovered that fathers talked to their children an average of only eight minutes a day on weekdays. Mothers did only slightly better, managing eleven minutes of conversation,' writes historian John R. Gillis in *A World of Their Own Making: Myth, Ritual and the Quest for Family Values.* Books such as Spencer Johnson's *The One Minute Father* and *The One Minute Mother*, with their formulae for the 'one minute praising' and 'one minute reprimand' might in a saner society be regarded as clever satires; instead they are snapped up as serious contributions to parenting practice.

As parents or children, we have unrealistic expectations of what family life should be like. Until the 19th century the idea of family meant little to people, except the rich and the aristocratic. Many parents often did not live long enough to see their children grow up. 'What is astonishing is that even children with two parents moved out of the natal house at a very young age in large numbers. Some did as mere children, but the greatest exodus happened in midteens, when virtually all young people lived and worked in another dwelling for shorter or longer periods of time,' writes John Gillis.

Families have always had to adapt to the larger social demands; for centuries parents had no alternative but to cede their rights to their children and indenture them as servants or apprentices. Families also reflect the current values of society and are not inured from the self-seeking, materialistic and heartless ethos of our consumer culture. Yet we tend to believe that the nuclear family as a safe, nurturing haven is the natural order of things and are disappointed and depressed when our own does not live up to that ideal.

TV can take some of the blame. Syrupy portrayals of family life have long been the norm in TV drama. For all its explicit language, even *The Osbournes* was a carefully sanitised version of family life. Real families are much more combative. There's nothing like a good (non-physical) scrap, say Drs Jeffrey and Carol Rubin in their book *When Families Fight – How to Handle Conflict with Those You Love.* The Rubins set out to dispel a number of myths about family life. 'Not only is it nonsense to perceive fighting as intrinsically bad, but it is also folly to ignore the potential for growth and change that can be a by-product. It is through fights within a healthy give-and-take atmosphere that family members get to test themselves, their boundaries, their peers, their children, their parents, to ultimately emerge with a sense of who they are.'

Fighting is inevitable in families and avoiding conflict isn't always healthy. 'The degree of coercion required to bring about family "harmony" can be very costly. Families and individuals within a family draw strength from the ability to tolerate differences, from learning that people can live together and enjoy one another, despite profound differences of values and outlook.'

That, of course, is a lot easier said than done. Family can be hurtful and damaging as well as nurturing and supportive. But it's a bond that mostly endures in spite of acrimony and absence. As the Robert Frost line goes, 'Home is the place where, when you have to go there, they have to take you in.'

EIGHTEEN

Stand by Your Man

'Stand by Your Man' was country singer Tammy Wynette's signature song, but if she had followed her own advice, statistics suggest she might be still be alive today. Married people live longer, healthier lives. Wynette married five times, and died at the age of fifty-five. People who place great importance on marriage, as Wynette obviously did, suffer most when their marriages break up. Evidence suggests that people who are divorced, separated or widowed face a particularly high risk of dying prematurely.

The effects of marriage on mental and physical health have been much studied. The evidence shows that marriage can be an important factor in maintaining health and living longer. How important? 'Marriage keeps you alive about three extra years, on average,' according to Professor Andrew Oswald of Britain's Warwick University. Professor Oswald and fellow researcher Chris Wilson cited the proof in a 2005 paper 'How Does Marriage Affect Physical and Psychological Health? A Survey of the Longitudinal Evidence.'

Their paper suggests that marriage is one of the best routes to happiness and mental well-being. A study of 17 developed countries found that financial situation was the best predictor of happiness, followed by health and marital status. Married people were happier than couples living together, who in turn were happier than single people. Other studies show that married women suffer less depression, and married men are less likely to abuse alcohol. The stronger your commitment to the permanence and importance of marriage, the more beneficial it is likely to be to your mental health (but the more depressed you'll be if the marriage breaks down). Men benefit most from marriage; women get more depressed about splitting up. Getting married again can increase your sense of well-being, but the effects are not likely to be as strong the second time around.

It's not clear why marriage increases our chances of living longer. It's known that isolated individuals have high mortality rates; social activities and friendship networks dramatically promote longevity. 'Marriage can be viewed as the smallest and most intimate of social networks,' say Oswald and Wilson.

One study found that the health of never-married and divorced men deteriorates 15 per cent faster than that of married men. Women, though, appear to benefit less. 'Controlling for socio-economic status and income, marriage offers a 20 per cent risk advantage to women, and much more to men. Unmarried males are 2–3 times more likely to die prematurely than married men. The protective effect is especially strong against "social" causes of disease [accidents, suicide, homicide or cirrhosis].'

It's not just living longer: married people enjoy better general health, get better sleep, have fewer visits to the doctor. 'Marriage may change lifestyles because of some kind of guardian effect, where healthy activities are increased and risky behaviours reduced.' If you're only allowed a puff on the patio, you're likely to smoke a lot less. Studies show that marriage reduces male drinking, though it is parenting that causes the biggest reduction in married women's drinking. Coping with shrieking toddlers when you've got a hangover is something you quickly learn is not worth it. Marriage is fattening for women and slimming for men, an Australian study found. The results 'show that, for women especially, there is a notable increase in body mass index associated with living with a partner ... In contrast, men have a reduced fat and energy intake in their diet, perhaps as an effect of the partner changing their eating habits'.

In a paper, 'Marriage and Public Health', American academic Maggie Gallagher cites a US Health and Retirement Survey that compared the incidence of disease in people in the fifties, who were married, cohabiting, divorced, widowed and never-married. The conditions included high blood pressure, diabetes, stroke, chronic lung disease, heart disease, psychiatric problems, arthritis, foot and leg problems, asthma, bladder and stomach problems, and disability. Gallagher notes: 'Almost without exception, married persons had the lowest rates of morbidity for each of the diseases, impairments, functioning problems and disabilities.'

So what makes marriage so health-giving? Gallagher claims that married people are more likely to look out for each other and act more responsibly. 'Cohabiters, for the most part, do not reap the same health benefits as the married do, because there are no shared social norms about how cohabiters "should" behave and because cohabiters typically have not made a permanent lifelong commitment to be responsible for and responsible to another adult.'

As a scholar for the conservative think-tank, Institute for American Values, though, Gallagher clearly has a political agenda. There is no logical reason why married and cohabiting couples, including same-sex unions, who have the same level of commitment to a relationship, should not enjoy the same health benefits. Many couples today feel they don't need the sanction of church or state to have committed and enduring relationships. (Indeed, up until the 19th century, many poor people never married but created their own informal rituals to exchange vows. The custom of wearing a ring, sometimes made of hemp or rushes, has nothing to do with Christian marriage; it dates back to unions in ancient Egypt.)

The longer the marriage, the greater the gains in health and longevity. But sticking with a bad marriage or relationship can have adverse effects. Psychologist Tim Smith and colleagues at the University of Utah conducted a study with 150 married couples. The couples were asked to discuss a subject that often triggered fights between them, such as finances or household chores. Their discussion was videotaped and analysed for evidence of hostility and controlling behaviour. The couples were also given a CT scan to check for deposits in the coronary arteries, evidence of atherosclerosis. The researchers found that the more hostile the wives' comments during the discussion the greater the extent of clogged arteries. Women who were in a relationship where both parties were hostile and unfriendly showed particularly high levels of atherosclerosis.

Hostility had no effect on the level of atherosclerosis in the husbands. However, husbands who displayed more dominance or controlling behaviour – or whose wives displayed such behaviour – were more likely than other men to have more severe hardening of the arteries. 'Another way to say it is that either being controlling or being married to someone who is controlling is enough to promote atherosclerosis in men,' said Smith 'So in couples where there was not a struggle for control – where it wasn't a contest – those men had much lower levels of atherosclerosis.'

A Swedish study found that women who report serious marital stress are three times more likely to be hospitalised for heart attacks or chest pain than women who report no marital stress. Other studies have shown that people in bad marriages have higher blood pressure, a risk factor for heart disease. Hostility in marriage has been shown to have other effects on the body. In one study, antagonism between couples was shown to decrease the release of cytokines, pro-inflammatory proteins that help heal wounds. On the first visit to a hospital research unit the 42 couples in the study took part in a discussion to help them support each other. On a second visit they talked about a subject that was their biggest cause of marital conflict. On each occasion, a blister wound was created with a vacuum tube on their arms and monitored for healing after their visit. The results showed that couples who were consistently hostile healed 40 per cent more slowly than others, with wounds taking an average of one extra day to heal. The study showed that production of cytokines was lower after the discussing marital conflict than after the support session. The research has more significance than the effect of hostility on the healing of wounds; changes in cytokine production has been linked to increased risk of diseases such as cancer, arthritis, depression, type 2 diabetes and heart disease.

All marriages and long-term relationships, of course, have their ups and downs. For many people, marriages improve after a bad patch. Problems don't always get solved, they simply go away. Money problems ease, children get older or less troublesome, a change of job creates a new outlook.

According to an analysis of the US National Survey of Families and Households, 86 per cent of unhappily married people in the late 1980s who stuck it out found that, five years later, their marriages were happier. Nearly three-fifths of those who rated their marriage as unhappy described it as either 'very happy' or 'quite happy' when interviewed again in the early 1990s. An Australian survey found that as many as 37 per cent of people regret their divorce five years later, and up to 40 per cent believe that it could have been avoided.

There's no question that a good marriage or long-term relationship is worth the effort. Economists have found, for example, that married people earn more money, a 'wage premium' estimated to be up to 40 per cent. (However, as any parent will ruefully affirm, they also spend more.) One study also found that the marriage effect on mental well-being is equivalent to earning an extra $100,000. And of course the general health benefits, already mentioned, are incalculable. 'For males, the longevity effect of marriage may even offset the consequences of smoking,' say Oswald and Davis. Instead of all those scary (and ignored) warnings on cigarette packets, maybe the message should be: 'IF YOU CAN'T QUIT, AT LEAST STAY MARRIED.'

NINETEEN

Be Wary of Your Pets

As a boy I had a pet white rabbit called Torchy. Torchy was usually kept in the garden, but on special occasions he was given the run of the house. One evening we had my sister Nuala's new boyfriend Denis over for tea and I insisted Torchy be allowed inside to meet him. The occasion went well until Denis got up from the dining-room table. 'Jesus, Mary and Joseph,' my mother exclaimed, 'would you look at that!' Mother was staring bemusedly at the bottom of Denis's right trouser leg out of which Torchy had chewed a large crescent. 'Sure, he just bought these,' said Nuala, unable to suppress a titter. Denis smiled weakly but I could see he was thinking, 'Fecking hell!'

Animals, ideal companions though they often are, can have a downside – and it's sometimes more serious than chewed clothes, scratched furniture or puddles on the kitchen floor. Pets can pose a health risk to their owners. If your budgie gets sick as a parrot, you could become infected too. If your cat has the runs, you could end up with diarrhoea. Give your turtle a cuddle and you risk salmonella poisoning. The medical term for diseases that can pass from animals to humans is zoonoses. People most at risk are those with compromised immune systems: AIDS sufferers, people on chemotherapy, the old, young children and pregnant women.

The common moggie carries several risks to owners. Ringworm is probably the most common zoonosis of cats. If you find yourself scratching red scaly patches of skin, it may be your cat suffers from ringworm. It's estimated that nearly three-quarters of normal cats carry the bacteria *Pasteurella* in their mouths. A bite from a cat may fail to heal and form an abscess. Antibiotics will be needed to clear up the infection. Toxoplasmosis, sometimes called 'litter box disease', is caused by a parasite in cat's faeces and may result in swollen lymph glands, rash, fever, headache, cough, sore throat and nasal congestion. Toxoplasmosis can cause miscarriage, premature birth or blindness in newborns. Pregnant women should not clean litter boxes. Recent research, however, may have men insisting that women clean out the litter box. Being infected with the *Toxoplasma gondii* parasite can cause women to be more outgoing, friendly and sexy, according to Sydney University of Technology infectious disease researcher, Nicky Boulter. (Caveat: a Polish study of women affected with *Toxoplasma* found they spent more money on clothes.) Men infected with *Toxoplasma* have lower IQs, achieve a lower level of education and have shorter attention spans. It's claimed that about 40 per cent of the world's population is infected with *Toxoplasma gondii*. Research also shows that infected people have a higher risk of developing schizophrenia and manic depression.

Dogs can pass on salmonella, toxocariasis, tapeworm, roundworm, *Pasteurella multocida*, *Campylobacter* and more. It's wise to discourage rough play with dogs and cats to avoid scratches and bites. Pets should not be allowed to lick your face or skin, or the cuts or sores of children. Puppies and kittens may look cute, but are more likely to be carrying diseases than adult animals. The incidence rate of *Campylobacter*, a gastrointestinal and blood infection, in kittens and puppies is as high as 42 per cent. Homebound pets are healthier than those allowed to roam and pick up bacteria from the soil or the carcasses of wild birds or other animals. Without regular de-worming of your cat or dog, you risk roundworm and hookworm infections, which are spread through infected faeces. Roundworms enter the body when ingested as eggs, then hatch into larvae. Though in most cases they cause no damage as they wander through the liver, lungs and other organs, they can damage tissue and affect nerves or lodge in the eye. Permanent nerve or eye damage can result. Hookworms move under the skin causing inflammation, but can sometimes penetrate deeper causing serious damage to intestines and other organs.

Petting zoos also pose risks. Children love to pet or feed animals, but animal fur, hair, skin and saliva can be infected with pathogens such as *E. Coli*, *Salmonella* and *Campylobacter*. These are easily passed to children who largely live a hand-to-mouth existence. Though petting zoos have hand-washing facilities, one observational study found that only 62 per cent of people used them. It's not necessary to touch an animal to pick up an infection. At a Colorado zoo, 65 people, mostly children, were infected with *Salmonella* after touching the wooden barrier around a Komodo dragon exhibit.

Would you be safer with a budgie or a parrot? Well, maybe if they're stuffed. Among the bird diseases than can be transmitted from bird to man are: *Mycobacterium avium complex* (MAC), psittacosis (parrot fever), *Salmonella* and allergic alveolitis. MAC is a similar disease to tuberculosis and is a lifelong infection that is reactivated when the immune system deteriorates. Psittacosis produces flu-like symptoms and is usually accompanied by a dry cough. It can be caught multiple times. (The textbook, *Viral and Bacterial Zoonosis*, records that 'in one incident 26 people who entered a room containing apparently healthy parrots contracted psittacosis and five of them died'.) Allergic alveolitis produces coughing and difficulty with breathing. The diseases are transmitted by direct contact with faeces or nasal discharges or by breathing in dried powdered droppings

And don't overlook goldfish. People with weak immune systems should avoid cleaning fish tanks. They can get very sick from a bacterium called *Mycobacterium* found in aquarium water. More and more exotic animals are being kept as pets, snakes, iguanas and other reptiles, all of which carry bacteria such as *Salmonella*. Monkeys are popular. About 80 to 90 per cent of all macaque monkeys are infected with Herpes B-virus or Simian B, a virus that is harmless to monkeys but often fatal in humans.

It must be said, though, that for people with normal immune systems the risk of catching a disease from your pet is small and is easily outweighed by the benefits of pet ownership, which may include uncritical acceptance and devotion – well worth risking sickness for. However, the number of diseases transmitted by animals appears to be increasing as human populations increase and have closer contact with animals. Rats, bats, mice, squirrels, pheasants, prairie dogs, geese, crabs, skunks, raccoons, guinea pigs, great horned owls, and pigeons are just some of the species to be wary of. The diseases you can catch from animals number in the hundreds. But that's nothing compared to what you can pick up from people.

World

How is it possible to find meaning in a finite world, given my waist and shirt size?

WOODY ALLEN
US MOVIE ACTOR, COMEDIAN AND DIRECTOR (1935–)

TWENTY

Take Your Glasses to the Supermarket

In the supermarket I watched a man get out a magnifying glass and study the label on a can. 'Always read the fine print' we used to be warned when dealing with secondhand car salesmen or loan sharks. Now it's the standard advice of every nutritionist. What have they done to our food that has made us so wary and untrusting? Nor is it just processed food that leaves us anxious. Fruit and vegetables, meat and dairy are also under suspicion: harbourers of pesticides, carriers of deadly bacteria, frankenfoods.

It wasn't always like this. Up until the 1960s, we scoffed without qualm mountains of meat and guiltlessly munched through plates of homemade cakes, cream sponges, biscuits. What fruit and vegetables we ate were often from our own gardens or from the corner greengrocer. But new technology that was developed during World War II to feed the troops was about to change all that. America, as usual, led the way. As Laura Shapiro says in her book *Something From the Oven*, 'the [food] industry came out of the war capable of feeding the entire world with frozen, canned, and dehydrated food'. The trouble was that many women were reluctant to give up what they regarded as a vital part of their identity – cooking for their families. A lot of food industry money, guile and effort went into changing attitudes to convenience foods. One of the tricks was to make it not appear too easy. Though instant cake mixes had been around since the 1930s, women were still baking from scratch. It was only when the dehydrated eggs were removed and women were able to add fresh eggs to the batter, giving them a sense of ownership, that instant cake mixes became popular.

Convenience we now know came at a price. Along the way we have become detached from our food and suspicious of its content. Now we squint at labels, fearful of every mouthful. Lurking behind every bite is a niggle that it's making us fat and unhealthy, slowly poisoning our children or morally compromising us through the mistreatment of animals, exploitation of workers or harm to the environment. Forty years of industrial food, health scares, and dietary somersaults have undone a millennia of untroubled and confident eating.

As Michael Pollan, author of *The Omnivore's Dilemma*, says: 'We find ourselves as a species almost back where we started: anxious omnivores struggling once again to figure out what it is wise to eat. Instead of the wisdom of a cuisine, or even the wisdom of our senses, we rely on expert opinion, advertising, government food pyramids, and diet books and we place our faith in science to sort out what culture once did with more success.'

Constant diet swings (low fat, low carbs and back), choosing food by fat or sugar content instead of relying on our sense of smell and taste, the endless negotiation with ourselves over what we can or can't have is forcing us into an unhealthy relationship with food.

It's no wonder psychologists are having a field day

analysing our relationship with eating. Food has always had huge cultural significance for humans, but our relationship with food has never been this dysfunctional. Food is our fuel, our medicine, our comforter, our enemy, our seducer, but rarely these days our unalloyed pleasure. It's also a yardstick with which we judge the social status and moral worth of others. In a revealing experiment, college students were asked their opinions of the morals of two Jennifers, fictional women of the same age, weight and attractiveness. One Jennifer had a preference for fruit, wholemeal bread, chicken and potatoes. The other enjoyed steak, hamburgers, fries, donuts and ice-cream. The first Jennifer was considered likely to be sexually monogamous while the 'bad food' Jennifer was seen as sexually promiscuous.

And it's here where our anxiety starts each week – the supermarket. It's no coincidence that no matter what supermarket you enter you find yourself first among the flowers and fresh produce. The message is 'Fresh and Natural' to belie the fact that most supermarket goods are anything but: shelf-life is often chemically extended for months, even years. Another curious thing. Despite the flowers, the apples, the oranges, the myriad foods all under one huge roof, there is hardly any smell. With everything chilled or hermetically sealed, appearance is paramount. We shop by eye.

We're hardly through the door before the angst starts. How many times have I met my Five A Day quota this week? In go the carrots, apples, tomatoes, bananas, cucumber – and the pesticides. In the scale of health worries, though, pesticides are hardly a cause for unease. The pesticides that plants naturally produce to ward off insects far exceeds the synthetic ones environmentalists warn against. A bigger concern is the estimated 26 million human pesticide poisonings, with 220,000 fatalities that occur annually, mainly among agricultural workers and child labourers in the developing world, and the damage to animal life and the environment. Consumer demand for cheap, blemish-free fruit and vegetables in our supermarkets has led to indiscriminate pesticide use, killing and injuring millions and polluting the world's waterways. Not something many people want on their consciences. And guilt is bad for your health. Research shows it can lower levels of immunoglobulin A, which are associated with a strong immune system, and can contribute to stress, depression and other illnesses.

Buying fruit and vegetables in the supermarket often feels like a duty. Didn't it once all taste so much better? It may not be nostalgia. Flavour is the last concern of supermarket growers; produce is selected for appearance, speed of growth and the ability to ship over long distances. Crops are picked unripe and are ripened artificially or stored for months. Fresh organic produce is likely to taste better because slower growth, thicker cell walls and less water produces more concentrated flavours.

.   Going organic will not necessarily make us any healthier, but it could ease our conscience, especially at the meat counter. Pigs, hens and cattle now lead miserable, unnatural, disease-prone lives before their body parts are turned into the bloodless slabs of protein that end up in our supermarket trolleys. That's not to say we shouldn't eat animals. As Pollan says, 'What's wrong with eating animals is the practice, not the principle: Industrial animal agriculture is ethically untenable.'

And not always very healthy. Most of the world production of antibiotics is now fed to factory-farmed animals as growth promoters and to limit the spread of disease in the unsanitary conditions in which they are raised. 'The antibiotics kill most salmonella, campylobacter and other pathogens, but spare the resistant strains, which then grow and reproduce. The manure from the farms contaminates earth and ground water, and is spread through rivers into drinking water. Multiple Drug Resistance of bacteria is now a burgeoning danger in hospitals and claiming many lives,' says scientist Walter Gratzer in his history of nutrition, *Terrors of the Table*.

As Gratzer points out, though, our food is a great deal safer than in the past when there was little government regulation. In the 19th century, blood and pus from diseased cows was common in milk. It was also half watered-down with flour added and pulped calves' brains to simulate cream. Adulteration was common in many foods. Lead acetate in wine, iron filings in tea leaves, machine oil in salad oil, sheep's intestines in beer, mercury in confectionery and, incredibly, grated umbrella handles sold as Parmesan cheese.

Today adulteration is much more sophisticated and pervasive. While there is little evidence that additives, preservatives, antioxidants, sweeteners, emulsifiers, thickeners, gelling agents, acidity regulators, anti-caking agents, anti-foaming agents, humectants, modified starches, and propellants in our foods are doing us harm, most, apart from preservatives, haven't been added for the good of our health.

The benefit of modern food adulteration, though, is that you can read about it on the label. Take a look at this packet of chicken rice. It's got flavour enhancer (621), antioxidant (320), emulsifier (471), food acid (270), flavour enhancer (631, 627) – and about 30 more ingredients. Decoded, flavour enhancer 621 is MSG, antioxidant 320 is butylated hydroxyanisole, emulsifier 471 is mono- and di-glyerides of fatty acids, food acid 270 is lactic acid . . . Could this be why supermarkets are now open 24 hours?

Even when it's in plain English, it doesn't necessarily mean what it says. 'Made from natural' indicates that the manufacturer started from a natural source but it may have been heavily processed along the way. 'No Added Sugar' – we've saved money because there's more than enough natural sugar here. 'Enriched' is a warning the food wasn't very nutritious in the first place. 'Fruit drink' may be no more than sugar and water with added vitamin C. Low fat is not the same as low calorie: sugar might have been substituted for the fat. Nor can we rely on healthy eating endorsements from groups such as the Heart Foundation. Food manufacturers have to pay hefty sums to have their products endorsed, so they may not be the healthiest in their food group.

To be fair to supermarkets, a lot of our anxiety about food is fuelled by the plethora of health experts telling us what we ought or ought not to eat. But the link between diet and health is uncertain and confusing. For example, Harvard researchers, using data from the famed Framingham Heart Study, found that restricting fat might help prevent a heart attack but increase your risk of stroke. Studies have shown that a lifetime of avoiding saturated fats is hardly worth the effort; it may increase life expectancy in a healthy person by anything from three days to four months. There is little or no scientific evidence to suggest a link between cancer and diet. The case for a blanket restriction on salt is not justified when studies show that it raises blood pressure only in some people some of the time. Sugar has been demonised, yet the only solid scientific evidence against it is that it can cause tooth decay but not as fast as those little packs of raisins mothers dole out to kids. As for fibre, evidence now suggests it does not prevent bowel cancer but it does reduce the body's uptake of calcium – not good news if you're worried about osteoporosis.

All the studies that link certain diets with good health are observational and, as consumers are only too well aware, dietary advice may change tomorrow. As Felipe Fernandez-Armesto observed in his *Food: A History*: 'Dietitians like to cultivate a "scientific self image", stripped of any cultural context. But they are children of their times and legatees of long tradition. Dietary obsession is a fluctuation of cultural history, a modern disease, of which no health food can cure us.'

Maybe we need to forget about the fat, salt or sugar content and focus on the overall quality of our food. Salt, for example, may not be the demon that health educators claim, but it's still worth avoiding. It's liberally added to processed food because it binds with water and increases the weight so you pay more. It makes synthetic food taste more flavoursome and encourages you to eat more. And it's the *more* that may be affecting our health rather than individual ingredients.

The French and Italians eat all sorts of decadent food that would bring the average dietitian out in a sweat: thick cream and butter, high-fat cheeses, salamis, pork sausages, lard, calorie-packed chocolate desserts. But they have a food culture that's based on quality not quantity. Eating is also a social occasion, not a refuelling in front of the TV. We tend to eat less when we share a meal with others. Continental food culture seems to pay health dividends. A study by scientists at Leicester University found that though life expectancy is fairly similar across Europe, Italians stay healthier for longer. An Italian man can expect to stay healthy 10 years longer than his British counterpart, and an Italian woman enjoys 14 years more good health than a British woman. Italians are not paralysed by food fear; they spend more of their income on good food and spend more time preparing and enjoying it.

In contrast, the British, for example, average less than 15 minutes preparing food; in the 1930s they used to spend three hours. Sure, most people are busier now, but advertising has worked hard to sell us convenience foods and portray daily meal preparation as drudgery. Cooking has now become a hobby, something we dabble in at the weekend under the tutelage of the latest TV celebrity chef.

All that TV food snobbery and gastroporn, though, does seem to be eroding our acceptance of processed supermarket food. The growth of farmers' markets in the US, Britain and Australasia shows that some consumers at least are hungry for fresh, locally grown, seasonal, tasty food and human interaction that extends beyond an obligatory flash of eye contact and a bored 'How's yer day been so far?'

But escaping from the food aisles may not be as easy as we think. Are we, as one writer has suggested, bonded to the supermarket in a consumer version of the Stockholm Syndrome? Dependent on our captors to the point of not trusting outsiders, we seek help from the very people who have turned us into dysfunctional eaters in the first place. Indeed, one British government survey found that consumers in their early twenties were reluctant to use greengrocers, butchers or farmers' markets because 'they express anxiety about entering environments that do not have pre-packed produce available'.

In Britain, some supermarkets are trying to make their stores more engaging and personal, with in-store Starbucks outlets and nail bars. Tesco provides own brand DIY Separation and Divorce Kits and, no reflection on their food, Last Will and Testament CD ROMs. ASDA, the British subsidiary of Wal-Mart, now employs 160 chaplains to roam the aisles of its supermarkets, a friendly face at the bakery for the spiritually bewildered, a word of advice to the young by the cereals. *Lettuce pray. Forgive us our dietary sins and set us on the path of nutritional salvation. Frozen Lamb of God, have mercy on us.*

TWENTY-ONE

Work to Live

When slavery was abolished throughout the British Empire in 1834, it created a dilemma for business. How could the new autonomous workers be induced to labour just as hard when they could maintain their simple way of life by earning a pittance and enjoy the rest of the week lazing in the sun? As Noam Chomsky says in his book *501*, a solution had already been worked out. 'As abolition was being prepared, a British Parliamentarian observed (1833) that "To make them labour, and give them a taste for luxuries and comforts, they must be gradually taught to desire those objects which could be attained by human labour. There was a regular progress from the possession of necessaries to the desire of luxuries; and what once were luxuries, gradually came . . . to be necessaries. This was the sort of progress the Negroes had to go through, and this was the sort of education to which they ought to be subject in their period of probation."'

The truth is that, for most of human history, people did only enough work to get by. Working for others, and physical labour, was frowned upon, something you did only if you had to. Craftsmen and craftswomen worked until they had enough money to enjoy the rest of the week in the tavern or playing games. Even on the days they did work, they kept their own hours, starting late or taking long lunch breaks. 'Life in the pre-industrial days was a bit like the life of a college student – irregular eating and sleeping, intermingled with intense drinking, partying, and all-night work sessions,' writes sociologist Joanne B. Cuilla in her book, *The Working Life: The Promise and Betrayal of Modern Work*.

Where did we go wrong? Life in the 21st century is a monastic regime of endless harried work from daybreak to dark, a treadmill that our ancestors would have thought ludicrous and insane for people who enjoy a level of wealth unsurpassed in history. Americans now work longer than they did in the 1920s. The average British household (where one adult is employed) spent nearly eight weeks more in paid employment in 1998 than in 1981. And that's not counting the stressful hours spent travelling to and from work.

'Now people are working harder than their grandparents did, and a significant minority of the highest status jobs require the kind of hours which would have been familiar to Victorian millhands,' says Madeleine Bunting in her book, *Willing Slaves: How the Overwork Culture Is Ruling Our Lives*. Industrial reforms in Australia and New Zealand has ratcheted up working hours to among the highest in the OECD. In Japan, they have a word for working to death – *karoshi*; in China it's called *guolaosi*.

The effects of overwork on our physical, mental and social well-being have been well documented. A recent American study, for example, found that overtime and long work hours are linked with an increased risk of hypertension, cardiovascular disease, fatigue, stress, depression, musculoskeletal disorders, chronic infections, diabetes and other general health complaints. 'If you work consistently long hours, over 45 a week every week, it will damage your health, physically and psychologically,' British stress expert Professor Cary Cooper told the UK *Guardian* in 2005. Workers begin to suffer from a permanent condition of stress that does not go away even after four weeks' holiday. In Japan, one study found a U-shaped correlation between the average number of hours worked and the likelihood of a heart attack. Another study suggested that long-term job strain was worse for your heart than gaining 18 kg (40 lb) in weight or ageing 30 years.

What makes it even more stressful for the overworked is that they know that hard work is unlikely to count for much. The unwritten social contract that if you worked hard the company would see you right has proved to be an illusion. In the global marketplace, trust, loyalty and commitment – the big words beloved by business gurus – have turned out to be a sham; your fate is just as likely to be determined by anonymous shareholders in Tokyo or Wisconsin. (In *A Geography of Time*, sociologist Robert Levine argues that it is this insecurity and indifference to employees rather than long hours that affect health.) Nor is there extra compensation for the new job insecurity. The gap between executives' and workers' salaries continues to grow. CEOs walk away with golden handshakes even when they screw up, while the salaries of rank-and-file employees remain stagnant and they are jollied along with non-cash recognition, employee-of-the-month plaques, picnics, gift vouchers and cheap trinkets.

Meanwhile, more and more is expected as organisations 'strive for excellence', cutting staff but raising output. As Bunting says, 'Doing a job well is no longer enough; "stretch targets" deliberately push the boundaries of the possible; there are no limits to the expectations.' Employees are organised into teams, which has the effect of neutralising dissidents. Even the most reluctant worker will put in the extra hours to avoid letting down his fellow team members.

Mobile phones, text-messaging and email have speeded up work transactions and brought work into the home, lengthening and intensifying the working day. One engineer surveyed in the New Zealand Council of Trade Unions' study of the impact of long work hours on families reported that he had to have his phone on 'from 6.00 a.m. to 6.00 p.m. every day ... so you haven't even started work and the boss will be on the phone talking to you; he does the same on the way home'. Another worker, a bank teller, told how her weekend free-time was gobbled up by bank-sponsored community activities such as cleaning up the local park. The work was supposedly 'voluntary', but regarded by the bank as essential for team-building.

It doesn't matter how disgruntled employees become though. As Cuilla says, 'Organisations no longer need to rely on people having a moral commitment to work. Shopping malls, debt and the advertising industry whip everyone, even moody teenagers, into obedient workers and customers.'

Toxic work spills into the rest our life, spoiling leisure time. 'When work is dull, tiresome or stressful, people are sometimes unable to do anything satisfying in their leisure,' says Cuilla. 'The more time demands of work dominate our lives, the more all activities seem like work. The clock and the schedule rob our social life of spontaneity. It is becoming rare for people to drop into a friend's house unannounced. We assume our friends are busy at home and don't want to be disturbed. When you are constantly pressed for time, home entertaining feels like work rather than an enjoyable leisure activity.' As work eats up more of our time, home life becomes more chaotic and disorganised. 'No one wants to be reminded of the daily tidying up, cleaning and repair because no one is doing it, and the list of chores never gets smaller. Our home becomes a reproach to us,' says Bunting. Ironically, we may come to welcome escape to the relative orderliness and calm of the workplace.

All this extra work also means the fabric of society and the community is wearing increasingly thin. The ancient Greeks observed that manual labourers make bad friends and bad citizens because they have no time to fulfil the responsibilities of friendship and citizenship. Many of us have even less free time now. Community groups, the glue that holds society together, struggle to recruit volunteers for their essential work.

A lot of paid work is demeaning, valueless and dehumanising. It's simply not worth doing for its own sake. As Richard Sennett points out in his book, *The Culture of the New Capitalism*, the emphasis is now on superficiality and speed. Sennett cites as an example computer programmers frustrated in their efforts to do a good job because the company is intent on shipping incompletely coded software, relying on consumers to pick up the bugs, thus creating a market for further versions. The more savvy employees now realise that careers are not about doing good work, but about promoting themselves as a 'brand' within an organisation. As Sennett says, in a fast-changing world being seen as having 'potential' is more important than past achievements.

If long work hours and sacrifice of family and personal time ever made any sense, it makes none at all now. 'This is an era when life should be filled with all sorts of rewarding activities. Yet many find themselves caught up not only in long hours of work but in debt, and suffering from stress, loneliness and crumbling families. Why? In part because we always want more, in part because we don't realise that we have choices,' says Cuilla.

We should heed the caution of Ronald Reagan who dozed his way through two terms as US President and famously remarked: 'It's true hard work never killed anybody, but I figure, why take the chance?'

TWENTY-TWO

Tune Into the Weather

Sometimes the in-your-face bonhomie of TV weather presenters is enough to bring on a bilious attack. But it's the weather, not its presenters, that usually affects your health. Human biometeorology, the study of the influence of the weather and climate on human health, is now an acknowledged branch of natural science.

It's something arthritis sufferers are painfully aware of. Many believe they can predict the weather because the tissue around their joints reacts to changes in air pressure. It's not just sufferers of arthritis or sinusitis who are affected by changes in air pressure. It can make dieters feel pessimistic or optimistic by turns. A drop in air pressure can cause the body tissues to swell and bulge slightly outwards so that clothing can feel tight: high pressure has the opposite effect, making you feel trim. Sharp falls in atmospheric pressure can bring on labour in pregnant women.

The shorter days of winter are also known to affect health. If you're depressed, have increased appetite, crave carbohydrates, need to sleep more, lack energy and are less efficient at work, maybe seasonal affective disorder (SAD) is to blame. In the Northern Hemisphere, up to 5 per cent of the population suffer from clinical depression during the winter months. Studies of animals have shown that seasonal changes affect the production of melatonin, a hormone secreted by the pineal gland in the brain. Melatonin is only secreted in the dark: light exposure acting through the retina causes rapid suppression of pineal melatonin. Though human melatonin is not suppressible by exposure to room light, bright fluorescent light can have an effect on humans. Light therapy – 30 minutes of sitting under a light box – has shown to rapidly treat the symptoms of SAD. Though SAD is not believed to be caused by melatonin production, the bright light therapy may be changing abnormalities in human circadian rhythms. Light therapy is being tried, with some success, as a treatment for circadian rhythm disorders such as jet lag, shift work and certain sleep disorders.

In Canada, where they have to take the weather seriously, a study showed that migraine attacks can be affected by weather. The study suggested that bad weather can worsen the severity of an attack in progress, while high pressure and clear sunny, dry weather had ameliorating effects.

Winter can be a dangerous time for the middle-aged and older, especially if they are smokers. According to one US study 53 per cent more heart attacks occur in winter than in summer and are more serious with a 9 per cent fatality rate. To combat the cold, blood vessels constrict to help conserve body heat. That increases blood pressure, putting strain on the heart. By contrast, blood pressure can drop by 10–15 per cent during the warmer months. Smokers have a greater seasonal variation in blood pressure and heart rate than non-smokers, and are at greater risk in winter. Winter is also a time when people tend to eat and drink more and exercise less. (If you need an excuse to take a couple of days off you could tell your boss you're suffering from Spencer's Winter Vomiting. This has been defined as 'an epidemic disease affecting both sexes and with onset at all ages, usually occurring during the winter months and early spring, and beginning in early morning. It is characterized by nausea, sudden and profuse vomiting, anorexia, constipation, pain diarrhoea and, less frequently, constipation, pale stools, headache, generalized aching, and fever.')

Diabetes is another chronic illness influenced by changes in the weather. The onset of insulin-dependent diabetes mellitus (IDDM) is more frequent in the colder months of the year. Whether this is because of increased viral infections or the effect of light on insulin action or hormone change or some other factor is unknown. Diabetic control is more difficult in winter, too, because people may be more anxious or depressed during the long grey months.

Diabetics often have poor circulation and so are more prone to common cold injuries like chilblains. Chilblains, patches of red itchy skin, affect women and children most. When exposed to cold, blood vessels – usually in the hands or feet – close up to conserve heat. When the blood vessels dilate with warmth, the skin becomes red and itchy, and blistering can occur. Chilblains can be irritating and painful. One old remedy was to dip the affected toes in 'the vessel under the bed'. Sticking your foot down the toilet, though, doesn't have the same folksy ring to it.

Spring brings its own misery for those who suffer from hay fever: sneezing bouts, nasal congestion, running nose, watering and itchiness of the eyes, nose and throat, and postnasal drip. For about 20 per cent of the population, spring is about as joyful as a visit from the tax man. Global warming is causing the pollen season to start earlier and last longer, and the effects of grass pollen are becoming more severe.

As pollen expert Professor Jean Emberlin told the UK *Guardian*, 'If plants are stressed by high temperature and/or pollution, they tend to produce more protein on the pollen grain to maximise their chances of reproduction. It is the protein content which is the allergen, which causes the reaction so the same amount of pollen has a more pronounced effect.'

Pollen does not usually exacerbate asthma because the pollen grains are often too large to make it into the bronchial system of the lungs and are filtered out by the nose and throat. But as the *Harvard Medical School Guide to Taking Control of Asthma* points out, there is an interesting exception. '[It] has been discovered in the mini-epidemics of asthma known to occur after a thunderstorm. It appears that thunderstorms create exactly the right climatologic circumstances to fracture ryegrass pollen grains into smaller granules of a breathable size and concentrate them in the air at ground level. These findings have helped researchers in England and Australia explain why patients with asthma needed emergency department care more frequently in the hours and days following local thunderstorms.'

The return of the warm weather is supposed to make people feel more sexy – but not necessarily more fertile. A 1990 study showed that both the density of seminal fluid and the sperm count are lower in summer than in winter. It's probably small consolation that dandruff production slows down during summer though hair grows faster, as do nails.

Summer used be considered a fairly healthy season, but that was before we became aware of the damaging effects of ultraviolet (UV) radiation and its role in the promotion of skin cancers. In Australia and New Zealand, overexposure to UV sun is particularly toxic because of the depletion of stratospheric ozone. UV radiation and sunlight have been implicated as factors in the development of age-related cataracts. A strong association has also been found between sunshine and mania. One study found that hospitals admit more cases of mania after a month of increased sunshine.

But not getting enough exposure to sunlight also carries risks of developing rickets and possibly cancer. Rickets was widespread in urban Britain and northern Europe in the 19th and early 20th centuries. The physical characteristics of rickets are distinctive and not easily confused with other diseases: stunted bodies with large heads, misshapen chests, twisted long bones, enlarged wrists and ankles, and bow legs or knock-knees. Puzzled as to why rickets occurred in some parts of the country and not others, scientists of the day eventually worked out that it was caused by lack of sunlight and poor diet. It was rife in industrial areas where coal smoke both from factories and domestic fires kept the sky overcast and children were often kept indoors away from the smut or played in sunless alleyways. In the countryside, and in smaller towns, rickets was unknown. Rickets is said to be the first childhood disease caused by environmental pollution.

Rickets results from a deficiency in vitamin D, a fat-soluble vitamin that is formed in the skin under the stimulus of ultraviolet light. Though some foods such as fish oil are rich in vitamin D, we obtain about 90 per cent of vitamin D from exposure to sunshine. Vitamin D enables us to absorb calcium and phosphorus for bone growth and for muscle and nerve function. If we don't absorb enough, our bodies leech calcium from our bones to keep our muscles and nerves functioning. Bones then become soft or deformed; in adults the condition is known as osteomalacia. Vitamin D deficiency can also accelerate osteoporosis, and is believed to increase the risk of certain cancers and diabetes.

The pollution that originally caused the epidemic of rickets may have gone, but the disease is making a bit of a comeback, ironically partly because people have been heeding health messages about slapping on sunblock and staying out of the sun. US vitamin D researcher Dr Michael Holick has estimated that 'a minimum of 25 per cent of adolescents and adults' in the US are vitamin D-deficient. Dark-skinned people are particularly susceptible to vitamin D deficiency. Supplements can correct the deficiency but require care because vitamin D is one of the most toxic of vitamins when taken in the wrong dose. No amount of sunlight, though, will cause vitamin D toxicity because the body is able to regulate its own production.

Studies of UV exposure by US scientist William Grant have found a correlation between cancer deaths across the US and UV exposure. Grant estimated that lack of sunshine led to 100,000 people developing cancer and 40,000 deaths – four times the mortality rate from skin cancer. A UK study reported similar results. It studied the lifetime sun exposure of 355 men, about half of whom had prostate cancer. 'The quarter who got the least sun were three times as likely to be in the cancer group as the quarter who got the most.'

Not only brother sun but sister moon can also have an impact on our health, it appears. The moon, Robert Graves' White Goddess, has long been thought to affect human beings during its waxing and waning. Most scientists would dismiss that idea as, well, sheer lunacy, but there have been a number of intriguing studies that challenge that view. According to a study conducted by Leeds University in the

UK, the number of doctor consultations increase during a full moon. Another study conducted over a 22-year period by the Institute of Preventive and Clinical Medicine, Bratislava, Slovakia found that attacks of gout and asthma peaked during new and full moons. In a recent study, *The Lunar Cycle: Effects on Human and Animal Behaviour and Physiology*, researchers of the Polish Academy of Sciences found a link between the lunar cycle and menstruation and birth rate as well as links with hospital admissions for heart or bladder problems. Traffic accidents, crimes and suicides, they said, also appeared to be influenced by lunar cycles. A study by Georgia State University in Atlanta found a relationship between the lunar cycle and food and alcohol intake. The researchers reported: 'A small but significant lunar rhythm of nutrient intake was observed with an 8 per cent increase in meal size and a 26 per cent decrease in alcohol intake at the time of the full moon relative to the new moon.'

Perhaps, though, a stronger case can be made for the effect of wind on health and well being. The föhn winds that sweep down from the Alps across Central Europe have been blamed for a 10 per cent increase in suicides and accidents. The gusty chinook winds bring warmth to Western Canada but also a sharp increase in migraine headaches. The blustery Santa Ana that blows across California is notorious for the irritability it causes. In his short story, 'Red Wind', Raymond Chandler writes about 'those hot dry Santa Anas that come down through the mountain passes and curl your hair and make your nerves jump and your skin itch. On nights like that every booze party ends in a fight. Meek little wives feel the edge of the carving knife and study their husbands' necks. Anything can happen. You can even get a full glass of beer at a cocktail lounge.' It's an ill wind that blows nobody good.

TWENTY-THREE

Don't Be In It for the Long Haul

Sardines can travel snugly in a tin, but humans have fewer options. We come in all shapes and sizes, but airline economy seats have only one configuration: too small. Dogs are given more leg room on planes than humans. Regulations require that canines travelling in the cargo hold must be able to stretch and turn around in their containers to avoid circulation problems. By contrast, the minimum space for human passengers, regardless of size, is only 66 cm (26 in) between the back of the seat cushion and the seat in front – and that's before the passenger in front hits the recline button. Leg room has not only decreased, but seats have also become narrower, and the use of new composite materials has reduced seat thickness by as much as 40 per cent. Your chances of having an empty seat next to you have also dramatically reduced. Advances in computer booking systems and alliances between carriers have enabled airlines to maximise loads. The days of being able to stretch out over several centre-row seats are long gone. Count yourself lucky if you secure an armrest.

Elevator-like crowding is not only unpleasant, it can take its toll on your health. Lack of blood circulation can have disastrous consequences for some air passengers. In fact blood-clotting can occur in any situation where people are forced to be immobile. The phenomenon was first reported in 1940 among Londoners who were forced to sit for hours in air shelters during the Blitz. Deep vein thrombosis (DVT) has been dubbed 'economy class syndrome', but a Dutch study published in the *Lancet* showed that immobility may not be the only factor likely to bring on the condition after a long flight. The researchers studied the effects of remaining sedentary in a group of volunteers who attended an eight-hour movie marathon and went on an eight-hour flight. On both occasions they were asked to remain seated as much as possible. The researchers found that chemicals indicating clotting in some volunteers were present only after the eight-hour flight. Low cabin pressure and a low oxygen level, the researchers suspect, were the factors that made the difference, not just the lack of movement.

Not all blood clots are life-threatening, however, and they only affect a minority of passengers. Smokers, women taking oral contraceptives, people with varicose veins, a family history of deep vein thrombosis or those who have had recent surgery are most at risk. DVT, though, can usually be avoided by taking low-dose aspirin for two or three days before a flight, wearing flight socks and getting as much in-flight exercise as possible. Contracting your calf muscles by clenching your toes while in your seat can also help.

A greater health hazard may be the air passengers breathe during flight. These days, airlines save money by mixing fresh air with recycled air – air that has already been exhaled by other passengers. The air is passed through special filters to remove dangerous pathogens, though clogged or badly fitted filters may only be 50 per cent effective. Another way to cut fuel costs on such aircraft as the Boeing 747 is to turn off some of the air-conditioning packs during flight. In effect, this means that fresh air is only introduced every 12 minutes. A sneeze can introduce a million droplets into the atmosphere. A computer model developed by Pall Aerospace and Boeing shows just one cough can disperse 100,000 bacteria-carrying particles over 20 rows. Even talking or yawning can spread infections. Bacteria can also be spread through dust particles and skin scales lodged in seats and carpets. Up to 30,000 bacteria per minute per passenger can be released on skin scales.

Bacteria thrive in high humidity, viruses in low humidity. Both conditions are present in aircraft. At the beginning and end of the flight, when humidity is high, there's a higher risk of bacteria causing abscesses, sinusitis, bronchitis, and in rarer cases TB and legionnaires' disease. In-flight low humidity creates a climate for viruses such as colds, flu and pneumonia, and ear infections. It also increases the likelihood of headaches, allergies, fatigue, diarrhoea, nausea, dizziness and irritation or inflammation of the eye, skin, nose and respiratory tract. One 2004 study by Martin Hocking and Harold Foster of Canada's University of Victoria found that 20 per cent of passengers who flew on a 2.5 hour flight developed colds within a week. The Aviation Health Institute website sells a 'bugstopper' mask for long flights 'which filter out at least 99.95 per cent of airborne particles down to 0.6 micron'. At the very least it will discourage the tiresome talker in the next seat and scare off small children.

On high-altitude flights the humidity can drop as low as 1 per cent, drier than a desert. Your eyes can get scratchy and bloodshot, and your skin dries out. The dry air makes it harder for your respiratory defence systems to ward off infection. Unfortunately, beer is not a good solution for the inevitable dehydration. Having one or two drinks while airborne has the physiological effect of four or five in your local bar. A boozer's idea of heaven, perhaps, but on a long flight you may have to pay the price with a nasty hangover. To combat dehydration, air travel guru Diana Fairechild, author of the book *Jet Smarter*, suggests keeping a water-saturated cotton handkerchief over your mouth and nose for much of the flight. It will help your lungs and nose from drying out too much, and help block the spread of germs. Fairechild also suggests spraying your face with water from an atomiser or water spritzer used for ironing. Lubricating the inside of your nostrils with a vegetable oil, such as olive oil, will prevent the delicate mucous membranes from drying out and can prevent nosebleeds.

It may be wise to bring your own bottled water, though with new regulations this may be no longer possible on many flights. An investigation by the US Environmental Protection Agency found dangerous levels of bacteria in drinking water aboard 15 per cent of planes at US airports. Airlines generally serve bottled water to passengers, but often use water from the tanks to make coffee and tea, and passengers may drink or brush their teeth using the taps in lavatories. Flight attendants have been known to refill empty bottles of purified water with airplane tap water.

It's not a good idea to fly with ear, nose and sinus infections because the congestion prevents the air from flowing freely in and out of those cavities and can cause pressure damage. Seasoned travellers carry a decongestant like Sudafed in case they pick up an infection en route. Flying less than 24 hours after scuba diving is also not recommended because the change in air pressure affects other gases in the body. Low pressure onboard a plane can cause gas to expand in the stomach, causing bloating and, yes, farting. Fortunately there's a technological fix. GasMedic, a sort of anti-whoopee cushion, allows you to fart with abandon. As the literature puts it, 'The GasMedic flatulence filter backs you up two ways. First, an advanced fire retardant-grade acoustical foam minimizes the signature sound of each flatulence outburst. Next, a high capacity carbon filter absorbs and neutralizes the common odours associated with intestinal gas.'

Fainting is the most common in-flight incident, caused in part by high levels of carbon dioxide in the cabin. A study showed that fainting occurs more frequently when only 10 cubic feet per minute of air is available to passengers. In economy class passengers usually have to make do with only seven cubic feet, compared to the 50 cubic feet in first class and about 150 in the cockpit. With 25 per cent less oxygen to breathe on board, you shouldn't expect to get any serious work done because intellectual capacity drops off: you're likely to make more sense of Stephen King than Stephen Hawking. Attendants who have to move around a lot during the flight are likely to be the most intellectually impaired. One study found memory loss among UK flight attendants during flight. It should come as no surprise that the drink you asked for never arrives.

A plane is not a good place to have your next medical emergency, but planes are equipped with comprehensive medical kits including in many cases automatic external defibrillators, and staff have CPR training. Few people die in-flight – more deaths occur on the ground because of 'airport tumult': heart attacks brought on by lugging heavy cases, stress of delayed flights and other departure trauma. However, at least one airline, Singapore Airlines, has had a 'corpse cupboard' built into its fleet of Airbus A340-500 aircraft. The upside of having someone die next to you is that you get to spread yourself over two seats.

Flying can be an ordeal for the faint-hearted, the fat or the hypochondriac, but most people arrive at their destination grumpy and tired but unscathed. Jet lag is probably the most lasting effect you will have to put up with. Sunglasses worn during the latter stages of the flight and for the first couple of hours on the ground can offset the effects of jet lag, according to Dr Chris Idzikowski, director of the Edinburgh Sleep Centre that conducted a study on jet lag for British Airways. However if your name is Mohamed or Khalid, sunglasses may not be a good idea.

Flying is never going to be a pleasant experience, especially if you're destined always to fly cattle class. But it might be wise to grin and bear it rather than become a whiner. In *Air Babylon*, her exposé of the industry, Imogen Edwards-Jones offers this salutary advice: 'Flight staff can spit on your food, piss in your coffee and wipe your steak around the rim of the toilet before it gets anywhere near your mouth. And you would be none the wiser. Some of the more badly behaved cabin crew carry laxative powder that they use to spike the drinks and food of those who get on their tits. It's a simple form of revenge that it is not readily traceable. So the best way to get the best service is to be pleasant and affable from the off.'

TWENTY-FOUR

Try Not to Take
Globetrotting Literally

There's very little, these days, that you can buy on holiday that you can't get at home, but it's still possible to pick up an exotic disease. Guinea worm disease, leptospirosis, Japanese encephalitis, lassa fever, ebola and marburg virus, monkey pox, bilharzia, elephantiasis, chagas disease and Buruli ulcer are all guaranteed to make your doctor's day.

It's likely to be the more common hazards, though, that put your health at risk and spoil your holiday. A few years ago I arrived in Delhi during a heat wave. The temperature was hovering around 50° Celsius (122° Fahrenheit). From the window of my air-conditioned hotel room, though, it did not look like extreme weather. It seemed wimpish to let a bit of heat stop me from getting my first taste of the subcontinent. I decided on a trip to the zoo nearby. Within minutes of leaving the hotel, my T-shirt was sodden with sweat and I was feeling very uncomfortable. As soon as I entered the zoo, I knew I had made a mistake. The sun was like a blast from an open furnace door and there was no shelter of any kind. The one bit of shade, under a single dusty tree, was occupied by a couple of Indian families. I walked on briefly, not sure what to do. Then instinctively I knew I had to get out of the sun. Feeling panicky, I retraced my steps and took a taxi back to my air-conditioned hotel. I have never experienced such oppressive heat since.

Though I knew nothing about heatstroke at the time, I think I made the right decision. Most people have a greater instinctive fear of freezing to death than dying from heat, yet heat can have devastating effects on the body. Studies have shown that cooling the brain to 33°C (91°F), effectively inducing hypothermia, can significantly decrease brain damage after a heart attack, but there are no benefits to be gained by heating the body. By the time body temperature reaches 41°C (105°F) cells have been irreversibly damaged. An increase of only 5 per cent in the body's core temperature is fatal.

Heatstroke is relatively easily to avoid, but it's harder to deal with threats such as malaria. Malaria is endemic in large parts of the world, including Central and South America, Africa, much of Asia, Eastern Europe and parts of the South Pacific. Prophylactic drugs are not 100 per cent effective, and in some areas the parasites that cause malaria are resistant to common anti-malarial drugs such as chloroquine. However, if you're relying on homeopathic medicines, then you've got no protection at all. In the European Union in 2000, WHO statistics show 15,528 travellers returned home with malaria. Malaria can strike quickly and in the worst cases kill within two or three days of the first symptoms.

If you want to be absolutely sure to avoid rabies on your travels, you'll need to book your ticket to Antarctica: it's the only continent totally free of the risk. Rabies is caused by the bites of mammals, such as dogs and monkeys, but there are also cases of people who became infected after inhaling bat excrement in caves. According to Spanish neurologist

Dr Gomez-Alonso, you should also avoid rabid men. Gomez-Alonso has found that 25 per cent of rabid men have a tendency to bite others. He is convinced that the myth of vampires such as Dracula originated from human rabies victims. The vampire's sensitivity to light, its aggressiveness and hypersexuality are shared by rabies victims. There have been cases of rabid patients practising sexual intercourse up to 30 times a day, and 'men with rabies react to stimuli such as water, light, odours or mirrors with spasms of the facial and vocal muscles that can cause hoarse sounds, bared teeth and frothing at the mouth of bloody fluid'.

Fortunately, for the average fit and healthy package tourist, the most you'll probably suffer is a bout of diarrhoea. Contrary to popular belief, most travellers' diarrhoea does not come from drinking contaminated water. 'Dirty water can be a source, but it is much less risky than eating contaminated food. The risk of developing disease is related to the number of "germs" consumed, and bad food contains very large numbers of pathogens,' says Dr Jane Wilson-Howarth in her excellent book, *Bugs, Bites and Bowels*.

Eating in your four-star hotel is no guarantee that you won't end up with Delhi Belly, the Kathmandu Trots or the Aztec Two Step. Sizzling hot snacks from a street stall are safer then lukewarm foods served in the buffets of an expensive hotel. Salads are best left to rabbits; in some parts of Peru and Bolivia, for example, farmers break into sewerage mains and use untreated effluent to water their crops because water is so scarce. Ice-cream, even from an apparently hygienic supermarket, can be risky stuff.

Taking antibiotics to prevent diarrhoea can make things worse since the antibiotic kills off the friendly bacteria in the bowel, causing unpleasant and protracted diarrhoea. It's standard travel advice that you carry 'blocking' medicines such as Lomotil to cope with an attack of the trots. However, Dr Wilson Howarth disagrees: 'Diarrhoea is a good thing. It is a natural process of expelling poisons which cause disease. By stopping this process, recovery may be slowed.' The important thing is to take plenty of fluid – at least two glassfuls after each trip to the toilet. It's the dehydration that makes diarrhoea sufferers feel awful. Oral rehydration solutions taken with boiled, cooled water are best – you can make your own with two heaped teaspoons of glucose (or sugar) and a quarter teaspoon of salt mixed in a glass of boiled water.

Travel would be much more enjoyable if we didn't have to worry about bowels and bladder. If, as humorist Doug Lansky has noted with his book title *There's No Toilet Paper on the Road Less Travelled*, it's also true that even on the beaten track a clean public toilet is hard to find. Some toilets in Rome don't seem to have been cleaned since the fall of the empire. Romania has some of the filthiest loos in the world. If you get caught short in Madras, you'll regret not packing adult diapers. In China sales of adult diapers soar at lunar New Year as millions jam onto trains for the long journey home to visit family.

The worldwide shortage of public loos is starting to be taken seriously. The World Toilet Organization, set up in Singapore in 2001, is dedicated to making the world a more convenient place. The WTO has run World Toilet Summits and Expos from Belfast to Moscow, inaugurated World Toilet Day, and has set up a World Toilet College (WTC) to train 'restroom specialists'. It's certainly needed. Dr Philip Tierno, author of *The Secret Life of Germs*, has advised that if you have to use a public toilet, it's best to use the first stall as it tends to be the least used whereas the last stall, which is the most popular, is likely to have the highest germ count. If you're supple enough, you should flush with your foot and get out fast before the cubicle is filled with bacteria-laden airborne water droplets. Tierno suggests singing 'Happy Birthday' twice to ensure you wash your hands long enough. (This is probably better done silently to avoid the stares of other toilet users.) Use a paper towel for touching taps and door handles.

No matter how clean the public toilet is, though, some people just can't go. They suffer from paruresis, the inability to urinate in the real or imagined presence of others. It's estimated that about 7 per cent of people suffer to some degree from this disability. Nancy L. Pickering of the International Paruresis Association has pointed out that, though no research has been done on the long-term physical effects of holding on, 'what we do know is that not urinating for long periods of time can weaken the elasticity of the bladder, causing less muscle tone. The bladder then needs to empty more frequently, which begins a vicious cycle for the paruretic. Urinary infections in both men and women can result from the build up of bacteria that forms from not properly and timely emptying the bladder.' Bashful bladder can also cause sufferers to take in less fluids leading to dangerous dehydration.

In an age of package tourism, using a strange or malodorous toilet is often the closest many travellers come to a real adventure. Our mishap in a bog in Beijing makes a better take-home story than intimations of mortality on the Great Wall. Everyone can identify with the trials of bowel and bladder. Surely a themed travel book will hit the shelves shortly – *Incontinent on Five Continents: A Public Toilet Odyssey*. It would be hard, though, to cap writer Mary Roach's account of using a convenience in Antarctica: 'Another reason to be wary of ice-sheet outhouses: seals occasionally use the opening in the ice as a blowhole. While there's nothing inherently dangerous about a suppositorial blast of hot seal breath, it is, in the words of one shaken veteran, "a disquieting way to start your day".'

TWENTY-FIVE

Scrub Up

If you're a woman reading this, I'll let you in on a grubby little secret. A lot of men don't bother to wash their hands after having a pee. The hand that clasps yours firmly across the meeting-room table may have been shaking dry a willie just moments before. Some women – and men – might find that thought erotic. The more likely reaction, I suspect, is Yuck!

I can vouch for men's hand-washing habits from personal observation, but there is plenty of research to back it up. When asked in surveys, people always claim that they wash their hands after using the toilet, but observation studies show that it's not always the case. In a 2005 US poll, 91 per cent of adults claimed they washed their hands after using a public restroom. But of the 6336 adults whose behaviour was observed, only 82 per cent actually did so. Other polls have found that fewer than half of adults always washed after touching pets, sneezing or handling money. Only 64 per cent of men and 82 per cent of women report washing after changing a baby's nappy, and 23 per cent of adults said they regularly handled food without first washing.

As a society, of course, we're often oversold on the importance of cleanliness. As a parent, I sometimes look back with amusement at the lengths we'd go to try to create a sterile environment for our first child: bottles stored in sterilising liquid between use, nappies steeped in Napisan. Nothing got within an arm's length of baby that hadn't been sterilised or boiled. By the third child, however, sterilisation had gone by the board. There was no time for hospital-type routines. And no need, apparently, either. The new arrival thrived just as well, if not better than the others, with normal household hygiene.

The cornerstone of hygiene, though, is adequate washing of the hands. Even in our hi-tech age, the simple act of hand washing is considered to be the single most important intervention in preventing the spread of illness and infection. When you consider that every inch of the human body is covered with 32 million bacteria – on an average day your body is crawling with a total of 100 billion little critters – the odd wash and rinse of the hands doesn't go amiss.

Unfortunately a lot of hand washing is perfunctory. Observation of hand washing and drying habits, for instance, has shown that people rarely use blow dryers to ensure more than 55–65 per cent dryness and often wipe their hands on their clothes. Wet hands can transfer more than 70,000 microbes by touch compared to only a few hundred when dry. Many women apply make-up while their hands are still damp, spreading any bacteria left on the hands. Wearing rings also increases the number of micro-organisms on the hands. Paper towels are the most effective way of removing bacteria. Swabs taken from the flow nozzle and air inlet of hot-air dryers show that many dryers are health hazards. In one study of 35 dryers in locations such as hospitals and railway stations, 'at least six species of gut bacteria (enterobacteria) were isolated from the air flows of 63 per cent of the dryers, indicating faecal contamination. It is concluded that hot-air dryers have the potential for depositing pathogenic bacteria onto the hands and body. Bacteria could also be inhaled and are distributed into the general environment whenever dryers are running.'

It would be a mistake to assume that people whose jobs make cleanliness essential – doctors, nurses, food handlers – are more likely to be thorough in their hand washing. Studies show that educational programmes to increase medical staff's awareness of the importance of hand washing have been unsuccessful. One study reported: '... medical staff have an inflated impression of their own hand-washing performance which may possibly prejudice learning'. In 1992, the *New England Journal of Medicine* reported on a hand-washing study in an intensive care unit. Despite special education and monitored observation, hand-washing rates were as low as 30 per cent and never rose above 48 per cent.

If doctors and nurses are lax in their hand-washing habits, is it likely that the spotty teenager behind the deli counter at your local supermarket is a paragon of cleanliness? Don't be lulled into a false sense of security by those latex gloves. Studies on the use of gloves by food handlers suggest that the increased safety margin thought to be derived from wearing gloves may be grossly overestimated. Many studies have shown that vinyl/latex gloves have pre-existing punctures and tears or get ripped or torn during use – damage that remains unknown to the wearer. 'Additionally as one wears vinyl or latex gloves, the normal and contaminated micro-organisms are provided a more favourable environment (increased moisture, nutrients and warmth) to reproduce than is offered by bare hands,' observed one report. Unless hands are washed thoroughly before gloving, the risk of contamination is increased.

Our hands contaminate everything they touch. One of the reasons Donald Trump may never have tried to buy himself a term as US President is because he can't bear the thought of all that handshaking. 'I'm not a big fan of the handshake,' he once told NBC. 'I think it's barbaric, shaking hands – you catch colds, you catch the flu, you catch this, you catch all sorts of things.'

He may have a point. Louis Pasteur, the father of microbiology, who first theorised that contagious diseases were caused by germs, refused to shake hands. Ever.

Pills
and Ills

One of the first duties of the
physician is to educate the
masses not to take medicine.

SIR WILLIAM OSLER
BRITISH PHYSICIAN (1849–1919)

TWENTY-SIX

Learn the Difference Between
a Pill and an iPod

It's an immutable consumer law that the latest, coolest, most technically advanced and cheapest version of any product comes out a week after you bought the current model. As soon as you leave the shop with your snazzy new digital camera, another appears in the window with double the megapixels and built-in GPS. Competition means that most of what we buy is in a constant cycle of innovation. We've been conditioned to believe that newer is better because it's true for most things. But not for drugs. Despite the claims of drug companies, many new drugs are not any more effective than older cheaper ones. What's more worrying is that they may put your health at risk.

Public Citizen, the independent US watchdog group, 'recommends waiting seven years before taking a newly approved drug, unless it is a breakthrough drug, which is a drug that offers documented advantages in healing over older, proven drugs. Many new drugs have been taken off the market during the first seven years they were available, because they have proven dangerous to patients. By relying on older, safer drugs, patients can minimize risk.'

There's good reason to be cautious. Clinical testing of

new drugs is done with only a small number of people (about 3000 people in the US). If there are serious side effects, they may not become apparent until the drug is taken by 10,000, 100,000 or a million people. Drugs are now approved much faster than in the past, so testing is of shorter duration and the trials themselves are designed and sponsored by the drug companies. The results of clinical trials are, of course, what conscientious doctors rely on when they prescribe drugs. But how reliable is the evidence? The medical profession likes to present to the public an air of authority, but when you delve into the literature it's apparent that medical science has many rickety structures that do not stand up to close inspection.

It's disturbing, for instance, to read in a standard textbook, *Clinical Trials: A Practical Approach* by medical statistician Professor Stuart J. Pocock, that 'there is a tendency for students, and indeed many clinicians, to treat the medical literature with undue respect. Many journals such as the *Lancet* and the *New England Journal of Medicine* are assumed to present new medical facts which are not to be disputed. Such a naive faith in "the clinical gospels" is perhaps encouraged by the dogmatic style that many authors adopt so that the uncertainties inherent in any research project often receive inadequate emphasis in the study report.' Pocock says many trials are poorly designed, are often 'of grossly inadequate size', consciously or unconsciously biased, and produce false positives. Moreover, trials that produce negative results are rarely written up or appear in medical journals. 'This *bias against negative results* by potential authors and editors can seriously mislead the medical profession, particularly when several trials are conducted to evaluate similar therapeutic techniques.'

However, as Richard Smith, who was an editor for the

British Medical Journal for 25 years, has pointed out, there is no need to rig trials or suppress negative results. 'The companies seem to get the results they want not by fiddling the results, which would be too crude and possibly detectable by peer review, but rather by asking the "right" questions – and there are many ways to do this.' For example, you can make your drug appear more effective by trialling it against a low dose of a competing drug. You can trial it against too high a dose of a rival and make it seem less toxic. By comparing it only against a placebo you can avoid comparisons with competing drugs. You can have multiple trial end points and choose the most favourable.

As a result, drugs of dubious value are promoted to the public and to doctors as real advances in treatment. The hyped Cox-2 inhibitors, Vioxx and Celebrex, are the classic examples. Vioxx and Celebrex were touted as breakthrough drugs that were not only superior pain relievers but also stomach friendly, with a low risk of gastrointestinal bleeding disorders, including life-threatening ulcers. For many people suffering from painful arthritis they seemed a godsend. Within a year of launch the sales were hitting more than $2 billion. Subsequently it turned out that both drugs increased the risk of heart attack. Both drug companies, Merck & Co (Vioxx) and Pfizer (Celebrex), had known there were risks from early clinical trials but delayed revealing the information. In 2004 Vioxx was hastily withdrawn from the market after many reports of cardiovascular side effects; an estimated 140,000 heart attacks and 56,000 deaths have since been attributed to its use. Celebrex remains on the market but with a black box label warning consumers of increased cardiovascular risks.

No drug, of course, is entirely safe. Doctors prescribe them on the basis that the benefits will far outweigh the risks. In the case of Vioxx and Celebrex, however, the benefits were far from clear-cut, despite the marketing hoopla. The studies showed that the drugs provided no more pain relief than the traditional non-steroidal anti-inflammatory drugs (NSAIDs) that patients were taking. Nor was it clear how many patients were benefiting from using a Cox-2 inhibitor instead of an NSAID to protect against gastrointestinal bleeding and ulcers. Not only was the number of people who suffered side effects of NSAIDs inflated in media reports, but it turned out the Cox-2 inhibitors were not preventing as many incidents of gastrointestinal bleeding and ulcers as first thought. A clinical study comparing Celebrex with aspirin showed that the incidence fell from 1.5 to 0.9 incidents per 100 patients taking the drugs for a year. Not enough, you'd have thought, to switch if you knew that you were then exposed to a higher risk of heart attack.

But there was worse to come. In *The $800 Million Pill: The Truth Behind the Cost of New Drugs*, Merrill Goozner takes up the story: 'A year after the study appeared, it [the *British Medical Journal*] reported that Celebrex's allegedly superior safety profile over the two NSAIDs in the company-funded study had been based on just six months of data, even though patients had remained in the study for more than a year. If the entire data set was evaluated, the Celebrex patients developed just as many ulcers as the generic and over-the-counter competition.'

Before embarking on a course of medication, which in the case of hypertension or cholesterol lowering may continue for life, it makes sense to establish what the real risks and benefits are. A pill that will reduce your risk of having a heart attack by 50 per cent sounds worthwhile. It makes a world of difference, however, to know whether it's a relative risk or an absolute risk. For example, if a pill is tested against a placebo and shown to increase survival rates over a 10-year period from 99 per cent to 99.5 per cent, it has shown a 50 per cent reduction in relative risk to the placebo, but the absolute reduction is a mere 0.5 per cent. It's basically meaningless, but drug companies will trumpet it as a 50 per cent reduction in risk and many doctors may prescribe it on that basis.

It's sometimes forgotten that drugs are fairly crude weapons, more akin to a shotgun blast than the precision strike of a laser. Antibiotics, given for an ear infection, for example, will also kill friendly bacteria in the intestines, possibly causing severe diarrhoea. Drugs are quickly transported around the body as a result of our efficient blood circulation system and can have a wide range of effects besides what we took them for. One British study found that taking popular heartburn drugs such as Nexium, Prevacid or Prilosec for more than a year increased the risk of a broken hip in people over fifty. As well as reducing acid in the stomach, the drugs may also make it more difficult for the body to absorb bone-building calcium, which can lead to weaker bones and fractures. Depression, dementia, insomnia, hallucinations, Parkinson's and sexual dysfunction are just some of the side effects from commonly prescribed drugs. Side effects often go undetected, especially among the elderly because the symptoms are written off as the effects of ageing.

A lot of harm may be done for very little benefit. Consumers who bought a new DVD recorder would be unimpressed if told there was less than a 50–50 chance that it would work when they got it home. Yet that's the reality with drugs. 'The vast majority of drugs – more than 90 per cent – only work for 30 to 50 per cent of people,' geneticist Dr Allen Roses told the British *Independent* last year. Dr Roses's statements raised some eyebrows in the drug industry, not because what he said is incorrect – the poor success rate has long been acknowledged – but because he is worldwide vice president of genetics at GlaxoSmithKline. While painkillers help about 80 per cent of people, only about 25 per cent benefit from cancer drugs, 50 per cent from rheumatoid arthritis drugs, 57 per cent from diabetes medication and about 62 per cent from antidepressants.

Despite all the medical advances of the past 100 years, medication is still largely trial and error. Though your doctor doesn't say 'Hey, let's experiment with this drug', that's what happens when he or she writes a prescription. Our genes determine how enzymes metabolise the drugs we take. If you metabolise drugs slowly, the standard dose may become toxic; if you metabolise rapidly, you may need a higher dose to benefit. Our unique genetic profile makes it impossible to predict whether or not we will have a serious adverse effect to a drug. Taking a lower dose for a shorter period can reduce the risk.

As Ray Moynihan and Alan Cassels document in their book *Selling Sickness*, a great deal of money and energy has gone into increasing drug sales by convincing people they have a medical condition or are at risk of developing one. Guidelines for cholesterol and blood-pressure treatment have been revised, lowering the bar and increasing the number of potential patients. Blood pressure of 120/80 used to be considered pretty good for an adult. Now under the US guidelines it is in the prehypertensive range, increasing the risk of developing cardiovascular disease. As Moynihan and Cassels point out, that increased the potential market by about 50 million Americans. 'As with the cholesterol guidelines, the high blood pressure guidelines were written by a panel riddled with major conflicts of interests. Nine of the 11 co-authors of the latest guidelines received speaker's payments or research funding from, consulted for, or owned stocks in a long list of drug companies.'

In 2003, writing in the *British Medical Journal*, Professors Nick Wald and Malcolm Law proposed that *everyone* over 55 should take a daily 'polypill', a chemical combo containing aspirin, a statin, folic acid, and three anti-hypertensives at half-dose. The aspirin would stop your blood from clotting, the statin would lower your cholesterol, and three anti-hypertensive drugs, a diuretic, a beta-blocker and an ACE (Angiotensin-Converting Enzyme) inhibitor would keep your blood pressure in check; the folic acid would be thrown in to counter a recently recognised risk factor, homocysteine. Based on a meta-analysis of randomised trials, the scientists say that 'changing all four risk factors together reduces IHD [ischaemic heart disease] events by 88 per cent and stroke by 80 per cent ... One third of people taking this pill from age 55 would benefit, gaining on average about 11 years of life free from an IHD event or stroke.'

But why stop at a polypill? Why not a megapill with an antidepressant, a diabetes preventative, and Ritalin to combat those senior moments? Even if a polypill did exceed all expectations, the belief that medication is the only answer because we are all prone to serious disease after age 55 would gain us nothing but a miserable and anxious old age.

TWENTY-SEVEN

Overcome Your
Cholesterolphobia

Cholesterol is a word that strikes fear into the hearts of the middle-aged. Like rust, cholesterol never sleeps; a gluggy buttery substance constantly seeping through artery walls, causing a build-up of plaques that any day now will block the blood supply to heart or brain causing a heart attack or stroke. It's that grim vision that's in the back of our minds as we tuck into bacon and eggs 'as a treat' or reach for a slice of cheesecake. It's that vision that chills us as the doctor says our LDH (low-density lipoprotein) is 'a bit on the high side', and our HDL (high-density lipoprotein) is too low. From then on, our life becomes a numbers game, a personal Dow Jones index of mortality.

Such is the demonisation of cholesterol that it's sometimes easy to forget that the link between cholesterol and heart disease is still only a hypothesis. No one actually knows what causes arteries to become blocked, and there are a growing number of researchers who are becoming sceptical about the value of lowering cholesterol. Leading the critical charge is Dr Uffe Ravnskov, a meticulous, independent Danish researcher and author of *The Cholesterol Myths*. 'People with high cholesterol live the longest,' asserts Ravnskov. 'This statement seems so incredible that it takes a long time to clear one's brainwashed mind to fully understand its importance. Yet the fact that people with high cholesterol live the longest emerges clearly from many scientific papers.' Nevertheless, a multi-billion-dollar industry is built on exactly the opposite hypothesis. In 2007, the global market for lipid-lowering drugs such as statins is expected to top $30 billion.

To a non-scientist, the cholesterol hypothesis does not seem very plausible. Cholesterol is not some toxic waste that builds up in the body. It's a vital substance required in every cell. It plays an important role in repairing and protecting the body. Without cholesterol our brains would be unable to function well: it helps us form memories and facilitates the uptake of serotonin, the neurotransmitter that modulates mood, emotion, sleep and appetite. It is a precursor of the steroid hormones that determine sexuality, and regulate sugar levels and mineral metabolism. Our liver manufactures about 80 per cent of the cholesterol we use, and diet accounts for the rest. The brain manufactures its own cholesterol because the lipoproteins that transport cholesterol are too big to pass through the blood–brain barrier. Cholesterol is also responsible for the production of bile acids, without which we could not digest or absorb fats. So is such a vital substance also an agent of disease and death?

There are many other questions that cast doubt on the cholesterol hypothesis. Why do coronary heart disease-related deaths occur when cholesterol levels are low, average or high? And why do men and women with the same cholesterol levels have very different rates of heart disease? It's also puzzling that some people who die of heart disease are found to have no plaques in their arteries and low levels of blood cholesterol.

The late Professor William Stehbens of the Wellington College of Medicine spent 50 years studying atherosclerosis, the hardening of the arteries, which is the underlying cause of coronary heart disease. He was a trenchant critic of the cholesterol hypothesis. In 2001 he published two papers, 'Coronary Heart Disease, Hypercholesterolemia' and 'Atherosclerosis: 1. False Premises, II Misrepresented Data', which put a large dent in the cholesterol hypothesis. As Stehbens has pointed out, atherosclerosis is a disease that affects us all: 'During the years from foetus to maturity atherosclerosis progresses when cholesterol levels are well below those allegedly preventing or inducing regression.' Cholesterol does accumulate in our arteries, but it is a manifestation that occurs as a result of the disease, not a cause of it, he argued.

Stehbens believed that atherosclerosis is caused by haemodynamics (the turbulent flow of blood). In the laboratory he was able to induce severe atherosclerosis in sheep by altering the flow of blood to mimic that in humans. The fact that as many as 50 per cent of people who have heart bypass operations go on to develop severe atherosclerosis again within 10 years seems to support this haemodynamic hypothesis. The recurrence of the disease obviously has nothing to do with cholesterol, Stehbens believed; it recurs because the grafted vein does not have the arterial architecture to support the increased volume of blood.

Other theories put forward for atherosclerosis progression include infection from a virus or bacteria that causes inflammation of the artery wall, high blood pressure on the artery lining, or high levels of the amino acid homocysteine, due to vitamin deficiency. More than 300 risk factors have been identified for coronary heart disease, including everything from obesity and smoking to baldness and earlobe creases.

It's cholesterol, however, that is endlessly promoted as the major risk factor of heart disease because there's big money in enrolling people in a lifetime drug regimen. Food manufacturers have also been quick to jump on the cholesterol bandwagon. Cholesterol-lowering margarines sell for up to three times the cost of standard margarines. Fat-free foods have proved a bonanza for supermarkets because they encourage consumers to overeat without the anxiety of increasing waistlines or cholesterol levels. Reducing saturated fat or cholesterol in your diet may do little to prevent fatal or non-fatal heart attacks. 'In fact, no clinical trial on reducing saturated fat intake has ever shown a reduction in heart disease,' says Dr Malcolm Kendrick in a Spiked (website) essay, 'The Great Cholesterol Myth'. Nor is reducing dietary cholesterol likely to be helpful. As the Framington Heart Study concluded: 'There is no indication of a relationship between dietary cholesterol and serum cholesterol level.' Ancel Keys, the American scientist most closely associated with the cholesterol hypothesis, put it even more bluntly in 1997: 'There's no connection whatsoever between cholesterol in food and cholesterol in blood. And we've known that all along. Cholesterol in the diet doesn't matter unless you happen to be a chicken or a rabbit.'

Drugs will lower cholesterol effectively, but the benefits of taking cholesterol-lowering drugs are not as clear-cut as drug companies like to claim. For example, in the 2002 ALLHAT (Antihypertensive and Lipid-Lowering Treatment to Prevent Heart Attack Trial) involving 10,000 participants, the rates of death, heart attack and heart disease were identical among those who took cholesterol-lowering drugs, statins and those in the control group.

Statins have been lauded by some doctors almost as magic

bullets, reducing the risk of coronary death by as much as 41 per cent. It sounds impressive, but when you look at the absolute figures, it is less so; some patients may well have second thoughts about embarking on a lifetime drug regime. The 41 per cent is taken from the 4S five-year study, which trialled the drug simvastatin (marketed under various names such as Lipex and Zocor). In the trial, 5 per cent or 111 individuals died from a heart attack; in the control group, 8.5 per cent or 189 died – which makes a risk reduction of 3.5 per cent. So where does the 41 per cent come from? By dividing the 3.5 per cent difference in risk by the control group's 8.5 per cent. To put it another way, if you have had a heart attack, the chance of avoiding death from another one over five years is 91.5 per cent; if you take simvastatin, the chance increases to 95 per cent.

When you look at studies of individuals with no heart disease but high cholesterol levels, the protective benefits of statins are even smaller. If you are about 55 and your cholesterol level is around 7.00 mmol/l, your chances of avoiding death from a heart attack if you take pravastatin for five years is 98.8 per cent. If you take nothing at all, the chance drops by less than one per cent to 98.2 per cent. Since statins have the same protective effect even when cholesterol levels are normal or low, it's hard to argue that the effectiveness of statins for people with heart disease is due to cholesterol-lowering. Some have suggested that statins' success may be due to anti-inflammatory, plaque-stabilising or anti-coagulant properties.

Taking drugs is always taking a risk. Statins are considered safe drugs, but since none of the studies have been longer than five years no one knows what the long-term effects may be. Some statins have been found to stimulate cancer growth in rodents, though the doses used in animal experiments were much higher than those recommended for clinical use. Of possibly more concern are reports from US cardiologist Dr Peter Langsjoen and others that statins can cause heart failure. Statins reduce the amount of cholesterol produced by the liver, but they also at higher doses deplete supplies of another chemical coenzyme Q10, which keeps the heart healthy. Deficiencies in coenzyme Q10 can lead to heart failure. The elderly are particularly susceptible.

In 2001, Bayer was forced to withdraw cerivastatin because of increasing cases of rhabdomyolysis, a rare disorder that causes muscle damage. Over 100 deaths and 1600 injuries have been linked to the drug according to Bayer. Statins can cause liver and nerve damage, mental disturbances, memory and cognition problems and a number of other side effects in a small number of people.

The US National Institutes of Health is conducting a study into the side effects of statins. While acknowledging the benefit of statins to men at high risk of heart disease, Dr Beatrice Golomb, who heads the study, says, 'However, benefit to survival with statins or other cholesterol-lowering agents has never been demonstrated in women (even those at high cardiac risk), in the older elderly, or in men at lower cardiac risk, and there are reasons to be concerned that the risk–benefit ratio may be less favourable in those groups.' As Golomb points out, after age 75 higher cholesterol is actually associated with living longer.

Many of the side effects may go unreported because some symptoms, such as memory loss and confusion, may be written off simply as old age. When Dr Duane Graveline, a former astronaut and aerospace research scientist, was prescribed a statin he found that after six weeks he began to have memory blackouts or transient global amnesia. In his book, *Lipitor: Thief of Memory*, he recalls one weird episode, 'In this extremely sobering experience with Lipitor-associated transient global amnesia, I regressed back to my teens for twelve hours.' A fate, surely, worse than death.

TWENTY-EIGHT

Keep Taking the Right Tablets

There are over two million medical papers published each year. So how do the general practitioners keep up? After a busy day in the surgery, do they curl up with a pinot noir and a pile of clinical journals, nodding till after midnight over articles like 'Double-Blind Comparison of Efficacy and Gastroduodenal Safety of Diclofenac/Misoprostol, Proxicam and Naproxen in the Treatment of Osteoarthritis'? Even if they were that conscientious, they could not manage to keep up with more than a fraction of developments.

Though many doctors are reluctant to admit it, studies show that much of their knowledge about advances in treatment comes directly from drug company advertising and/or 'detailers', (pharmaceutical sales representatives). Since the prime objective of any drug company is to sell their products in a fiercely competitive market, it's unlikely to be a reliable source of unbiased information. As well, some sales reps, driven by the need to meet quotas and the chance to earn huge bonuses, will go to almost any length to get doctors to prescribe their company's drugs. One sales rep posted this confession on the UK No Free Lunch website: 'As a rep, when you visit a doctor, you can't force them to sign on a dotted line that says, "I, Dr X, promise to prescribe your drug and no one else's." Why would he or she prescribe your drug when there's a cheaper, identical, but non-branded, version available? So you use every other tool at your disposal to persuade them – flattery, flirting, trips, expensive dinners. I used to come away some days feeling like an escort. I'm not saying I was expected to have sex with GPs, but I know some reps who'd sleep with doctors just to get their drug prescribed.'

Drug companies are increasingly using savvy, attractive young people, often women, to push their products. As the *New York Times* reported in 2005, cheerleaders are now being recruited to push pharmaceuticals. While some doctors are strongly resistant to sales reps, many see no harm in them. As bioethicist Carl Elliott wrote in an *Atlantic Monthly* article, 'The Drug Pushers', '. . . many reps are so friendly, so easy-going, so much fun to flirt with that it is virtually impossible to demonize them. How can you demonize someone who brings you lunch and touches your arm and remembers your birthday and knows the names of all your children?'

Drug-company marketing is incredibly sophisticated and thorough. Sales reps are taught to keep dossiers on the doctors they visit, with details of everything, from the names of their family members to their golf handicaps, to the foods they like or dislike, to the clothes they wear. According to one American ex-rep, 'Most companies have their own classification of the doctor's personality. One schema is that of the eagle-owl-dove-peacock, where the eagle is egotistical and domineering, the owl wants information and is very analytical, the dove is the friendly sort who gets on well with everyone and the peacock is a social butterfly/extrovert.'

The profiles enable reps to ingratiate themselves by adapting their own personal style to match the doctor's.

Obtaining information on doctors' prescribing habits, a key to getting them to switch drugs, used to be hard work but now, in the US at least, market-research companies offer that vital information for sale and it can be downloaded with the click of the mouse. Reps now know exactly how many of their drugs doctors are prescribing and if a doctor is lying to them.

Reps are often trained by role play using audio tape or videotape. They have a written script, which they have learnt verbatim and which can be adapted to different situations such as restricted time, personality type and so on. Visits to doctors are far from casual affairs. After the patter, reps get down to the all important 'close', getting a commitment from a doctor – 'Will you prescribe this product for the next three patients you see?'

To get to that point, sales reps may need more than glossy charts, facts, figures and clinical evidence. Free drug samples, pens, mugs, stationery, trinkets and food are standard inducements. In 2001, drug companies gave doctors nearly $11 billion worth of 'free samples', says Dr Marcia Angell in her book *The Truth About the Drug Companies*. As Angell points out, the drugs were not really free: the costs were simply added on to drug prices. 'Free samples are the most important gifts,' she writes. 'They are an effective way to get doctors and patients familiar with an expensive, newly approved drug when an older cheaper one might be better or just as good.' But, as Elliott says, the other freebies are important too. 'A particular gift may have no influence, but it might make a doctor more apt to think that he or she would not be influenced by larger gifts in the future. A pizza and a penlight are like inoculations, tiny injections of self-confidence that make a doctor think, I will never be corrupted by money.'

The temptations are real. Drug-company largesse is legendary. All-expenses-paid trips to sponsored conferences, cruises, lecture or attendance fees at seminars, and medical equipment are just some of the incentives doctors have been offered. Freebies often extend to receptionists, nurses and other practice staff, especially if the doctor is hard to get to. In his article, Elliott cites the example of former drug rep Gene Carbona, who 'arranged to buy lunch for the staff of certain private practices every day for a year'. Awash with drug company money to give away, he also once arranged a $35,000 'unrestricted educational grant' for a doctor who wanted a swimming pool in his backyard. Though these may be extreme examples, some doctors have come to regard drug company gifts as one of the perks of the job and are not above requesting sweeteners such as tickets to a sports event or concert.

Drug companies have found that one of the most effective ways to influence doctors to prescribe their product is to recruit other doctors to front seminars and lend their credibility to drug company claims. 'The semi-official industry term for these speakers and consultants is "thought leaders", or "key opinion leaders",' writes Elliott. 'Some thought leaders do not stay loyal to one company but rather generate a tidy supplemental income by speaking and consulting for a number of different companies. Reps refer to these doctors as "drug whores".'

Most doctors, though, are likely to have accepted no more than the free samples, the pens, stationery and other trinkets with the drug company logo and the occasional free seminar lunch. Most would probably resent any suggestion that their integrity had been compromised or their prescribing changed by such trivial attempts at influence. Yet study after study of the process of social influence shows that we can be easily manipulated to respond positively to requests. As social animals we have a strong natural tendency to reciprocate – to repay in kind what we have received. That's why supermarkets often have food sampling in store – it sells more products because consumers feel subtly obligated to buy. We also respond well to people we like. Good salespeople make a point of being affable, search for some connection between themselves and the customer, and never miss a chance to throw in a compliment. Doctors would be unusual human beings, then, if they did not respond to the drug sales rep's technique, sometimes called 'food, flattery and friendship'. And many studies show that visits from drug sales reps do change prescribing habits. A meta-analysis of 16 studies published in the *Journal of the American Medical Association* in 2000 concluded 'that physician-industry interactions appears to affect prescribing and professional behaviour'.

For patients it may often make little difference which brand of drug they're given, but if doctors are persuaded to prescribe more expensive drugs it will increase the costs of health services generally. That will mean higher medical insurance premiums and less funding for operations such as hip replacements in the public health sector. Inevitably, it is also the newest, most expensive drugs that are given the hardest sell, and drugs that have not been on the market long are unlikely to be the safest (see page 187).

Doctors may also be duped by drug company literature into prescribing drugs that are less effective or have dangerous side effects. As Angell has put it, 'To rely on drug companies for unbiased evaluations of their products makes about as much sense as relying on beer companies to teach us about alcoholism: the conflict of interest is obvious.' In the wake of the Vioxx disaster, the painkiller with side effects that caused an estimated 140,000 heart attacks and 56,000 deaths, documents made public in 2005 showed that the company directed its 3000 Vioxx sales reps to avoid discussing the cardiovascular risks involved in taking the drug.

Some reps may not even be aware that the drugs they are promoting to doctors may be dangerous. Reps are often the last to know, says Elliott. 'Of course for a rep to be detailing a drug enthusiastically right up to the day it is withdrawn from the market is likely to erode that rep's credibility with doctors. Yet some reps say they don't hear about problems until the press gets wind of them and the company launches into damage control.'

Over the past few years there's been a backlash against the excesses of drug company marketing and the use of what amounts to bribery and kickbacks. In 2000, the American Medical Association drew up guidelines to curb these practices and the pharmaceutical industry produced its own guidelines in 2002. No Free Lunch, an organisation founded to raise awareness of the dangers of pharmaceutical industry marketing among health professionals in the US, now has branches in the UK and Italy. In Australasia, Healthy Skepticism, a similar organisation 'aims to improve health by reducing harm from misleading drug promotion'. But there are huge incentives for drug companies to carry on what they are doing. As Angell has pointed out, the guidelines provide plenty of loopholes. Though targeting individual doctors is expensive, the returns are high. One study found that for every dollar they spent on sales reps, they recouped $10.29. In the past decade the number of drug company sales reps in the US doubled to more than 90,000. In the UK there are 8000 reps covering about 60,000 doctors, or one representative working full-time promoting to 7.5 doctors. There's no way of knowing if your doctor is prescribing under the influence. A visit to Worstpills.org for a second opinion could be worthwhile if you and your pills are going to be long-time partners.

The worst thing to do, if you have a medical condition that needs to be controlled, is to simply stop taking your medication. Surprisingly, however, that's what many people do. Patients' failure to take medication properly has been described as the number one problem in treating illness. Studies suggest that more than half the people prescribed medication for chronic diseases fail to take their medication, or don't take it as prescribed. One study found that 40 per cent of people being treated for hypertension, 55 per cent of people with diabetes and 80 per cent of asthma sufferers fail to take their medication regularly. In the US, it's estimated that medication non-compliance causes the deaths of 125,000 people with treatable illnesses every year. So, keep taking the tablets – just try to make sure they're the right ones.

TWENTY-NINE

Treat Yourself with Care

I'm awaiting with relish the day a drug manufacturer is sued for injury sustained while trying to undo tamperproof packaging 'triple sealed for your safety'. Don't they care that the majority us who attempt forced entry into a packet of pills are badly hung-over and liable to cause ourselves bodily harm with anything sharper that a spoon?

Unfortunately, opening over-the-counter (OTC) medication is not where the risk ends. It's often assumed that OTC medication is relatively risk-free. It may not be as powerful as the prescription medicine we get from the doctor, we reason, but at least it won't do us any harm. That's a dangerous assumption to make. Even a 'safe' medicine like paracetamol (or acetaminophen in the US) needs to be used with caution. Paracetemol can cause kidney failure and serious or even fatal liver damage. Studies have shown that even a small overdose of paracetamol, say twice the recommended dose, if taken while fasting can lead to liver damage. Drinking alcohol and taking paracetamol also increases the risk of liver damage. Taking just one paracetamol pill daily for a year doubles the risk of kidney disease. People prone to migraines or tension headaches who take painkillers like paracetamol more than three days a week could also end up with chronic rebound headaches and a drug habit that is hard to kick.

Coughs and colds are two of the main reasons we rush to the pharmacy, but recent guidelines released by the American College of Chest Physicians say we're wasting our time and money. There is little or no evidence that common OTC cough remedies are effective in relieving coughs caused by cold or flu. The panel of experts convened by the College warns against giving such products to children under 14 because they're more susceptible to side effects. Dextromethorphan, the suppressant used in products such as Robitussin and Vicks Formula 44, can cause agitation, muscle spasms and allergic reactions. Earlier-generation antihistamines, such as bromopheniramine, the panel says, may be more effective than the newer non-drowsy ones. Colds, like most minor ailments, of course, are self-limiting. By the time you get around to self-medicating, you may already be on the road to recovery, one of the reasons that ineffective drugs appear to work.

As the neighbourhood methamphetamine-maker will attest, pseudoephedrine, the active ingredient in many nasal decongestants, does work (and it's also the drug of choice if you suffer from priapism). But pseudoephedrine can have serious side effects. A simple cold remedy that contains the drug can cause blood pressure to rise to dangerous levels if taken with a monoaminine oxidase (MAO) inhibitor prescribed for depression. One man who took the decongestant Sudafed could not urinate and had to be rushed to hospital where the pressure on his bladder was relieved with a catheter. He had an enlarged prostate and should never have taken the medicine. Pseudoephedrine drugs should be avoided by people suffering from a whole range of conditions from heart disease to glaucoma; it can interact with everything from coffee to antibiotics, and can have a range of nasty side effects from irregular heartbeats to dizziness.

Most people don't think twice about taking an antacid. However, there's a danger that people with chronic heartburn may become too dependent on these drugs and not make recommended lifestyle changes, such as improved diet, to reduce flare-ups. People who feel they need to self-medicate regularly with OTC antacids may be suffering from more than heartburn; they may have gastroesophageal reflux disease (GERD), which sometimes develops into Barrett's Esophagus, a condition caused by long-term irritation of the oesophagus that can lead to esophageal cancer. Antacids that contain aluminium, calcium and magnesium can reduce the absorption of some tetracycline and quinolone-type antibiotics by as much as 90 per cent, rendering them almost useless against infection.

Some of the side effects of OTC drugs are listed on the packaging. But how many of us heed the labels on the drugs we buy? A survey conducted by the US National Council on Patient Information and Education (NCPIE) found that only 20 per cent read the warning signs when buying a medicine in the pharmacy and only 49 per cent bothered to read the usage information before taking it.

What makes those figures alarming is that more and more powerful drugs which used to be prescription-only are now available over the counter. The drug industry is pushing the concept of more self-care, i.e. self-medication, claiming it will be cheaper for the consumer and better for the health system, reducing the need for doctors to treat minor or routine ailments. In the UK, for example, low-dose statins can now be bought over the counter. While statins have been proved to reduce risk of death from heart disease for many people, they can have a range of side effects from muscle damage to memory loss. As a *Journal of the American Heart Association* article, 'The Argument Against the Appropriateness of Over-the-Counter Statins,' says, if people at low risk take them, then the risk may outweigh the benefits, and people at high risk of cardiovascular disease will not benefit from the low dosage. In addition, low levels of high-density lipoproteins (HDL), the 'good' cholesterol, may go undetected.

In some countries the anti-inflammatory drug diclofenac (Voltaren) is now available over the counter, though it carries risks of gastrointestinal complaints, which can lead to ulceration and bleeding, and in rare cases liver and renal damage. A recent study conducted by researchers from the University of Newcastle in Australia reported that it may increase the risk of heart attack and stroke by as much as 40 per cent. Direct-to-consumer drug advertising on TV, which is prohibited in every developed country except the US and New Zealand, builds an expectation that there is 'a pill for every ill' and increases the likelihood that drugs generally will be overused and powerful drugs used unwisely.

Generic drugs can be up to 80 per cent cheaper than brand-name drugs. Both have the same active ingredients, the same potency, are available in the same dosage and may well be manufactured by the same company, though the placebo effect will probably increase the more you pay. Doctors and pharmacists will tell you that it's best to throw out your expired medicines but there's really no scientific basis for that advice. There are exceptions – nitroglycerin, insulin and some liquid antibiotics – but the majority of drugs will be still be effective for years after the date on the packaging. Francis Flaherty, a former director of the drug-testing programme for the US Food and Drug Administration (FDA) told the

Wall Street Journal; 'Most drugs degrade very slowly. In all likelihood, you can take a product you have at home and keep it for many years, especially if it's in the refrigerator.' So why do most drugs 'expire' a couple of years after you buy them? 'Manufacturers put expiration dates on for marketing, rather than for scientific reasons. It's not profitable for them to have products on the shelf for 10 years. They want turnover.'

Drug companies don't dispute that their products last a good deal longer than the expiry date. By putting a two-year instead of, say, a four-year expiry date, companies are able to reduce any liability or safety risk. They also say that they don't want people using drugs they've had lying around for 10 years because the old package insert will not include the latest information or contra-indications. (However, the latest information on drugs can be readily accessed on the Internet.)

Drug companies don't usually test drugs to check if they are still effective after the official expiration date. It's only because of drug testing commissioned by the US military that we know for sure that drugs last a lot longer than claimed. About 15 years ago, the US military had a $1 billion stockpile of drugs, which if they followed the instructions of the manufacturer they would have had to destroy and replace every two or three years. They employed the FDA to test the drugs in their inventory to see if they were still useable. More than 100 drugs, both prescription and over-the-counter, were analysed for stability and potency. According to the *Wall Street Journal*, 'The results, never before reported, show that about 90 per cent of them were safe and effective far past their original expiration date, at least one for 15 years past it.' The FDA found that most drugs were 'surprisingly durable'. In one instance, drugs labelled for room temperature storage were kept in a warehouse for two years in Oman where the daytime temperature averaged 57°C and yet were still found to be potent after the expiry date.

No matter how 'expired' the drugs are, there is little evidence to suggest they will do you any harm if you take them. In 1963, one case was reported of kidney damage as a result of using expired tetracycline. This was supposedly caused by a chemical transformation of the active ingredient but that conclusion was disputed by other scientists. Studies show that expired drugs may lose their potency over time from as little as 5 per cent or less to 50 per cent or more, but even after 10 years most drugs have much of their original potency. There doesn't seem to be any justification for chucking them away after a couple of years if they've been stored properly

It's obviously better, though, to avoid taking drugs at all. To relieve minor ailments, it might be better to try a home remedy. Drinking lots of water when you have a cold may loosen mucus as effectively as any store-bought expectorant. Instead of taking an antacid for heartburn, you could try a glass of milk because milk proteins absorb the excess acids. The juice of a garlic clove with oil is said to be good for earache. A frozen gel pack or a packet of frozen peas applied to the head can relieve a tension headache. *The Doctors Book of Home Remedies* has over 1000 remedies for everyday health problems that doctors have tested and found to work.

Not that you're ever likely to get that sort of advice from your local pharmacist. Pharmacists like to portray themselves as helpful health professionals, but they're also retailers who are happy to sell anything that makes a buck. Most pharmacies, for example, now stock homeopathic medicines. There is not a shred of scientific evidence that these contain anything other than lactose and water. Homeopathic medicines are so diluted that not a single molecule of the active ingredient remains. The lowest dilution is usually '6X', which means that the active substance has been diluted and succussed (shaken) six times. This gives a concentration of one part per million. Many homeopathic dilutions, however, are '30C'. That works out at one part per 1,000,000,000,000,000,000,000,000,000,000 (yes, 30 zeroes). You could horrify friends and family by swallowing a whole bottle of homeopathic sleeping pills. The only likely effect is that the lactose (milk sugar) will keep you awake.

Homeopathy violates the principles of chemistry, physics and pharmacology – things you'd have thought 'health professionals' might have some regard for. Medicines work in relation to the potency of the active ingredients. The stronger the concentration of a substance, the greater the effect it will have on the body. That's not only scientifically sound but also simple common sense: a glass of whiskey is going to make you merrier than a glass of beer. Homeopathy, however, stands this principle on its head: the higher the dilution, the greater the potency of the homeopathic medicine. Homeopathy is claimed to be an alternative method of healing. But there is no 'alternative' system of medicine any more than there is an alternative system of car repair. There is only medicine that works – and there is overwhelming evidence that homeopathy does not.

Pharmacies are also happy to sell herbal remedies and dietary supplements of dubious value. Herbal remedies in most countries are unregulated so you don't know what you're getting because the strength and consistency of the active ingredients vary from brand to brand. It's also possible they may contain contaminants or undeclared substances. A useful herbal medicine like St John's Wort, for example, can vary according to where and how it was grown, the plant parts used, and how it was harvested, extracted and stored. Herbal remedies may also have dangerous interactions with other medicines (see page 234). Most pharmacists don't have any specific professional training in herbal medicine.

Self-medication is often talked up as 'consumer empowerment', but there's nothing empowering about paying good money for drugs, remedies or supplements that are not needed, may not work or could put your health at risk.

THIRTY

Read Between the Lines

Sometimes, but not often, what you read in the newspapers can be cheering. According to a news item, 'A Swedish study finds that people who use snuff are more likely to be overweight and to have high blood pressure and high cholesterol.' I've never been tempted by snuff, the fine ground tobacco you sniff between forefinger and thumb, so that's one less health risk I have to worry about. There was a warning, too, that guitarists could suffer a form of mastitis, caused by holding the instrument against their chests. Another study found that eating too many liquorice allsorts can damage a man's sex drive. Rap music, it's been discovered, can cause you to speed and drive dangerously. None of these risks causes me the least concern.

Unfortunately, they're far outweighed by the seemingly endless health risks of ordinary daily living. Taking a shower may cause brain damage because it could expose people to dangerously high levels of manganese, a poisonous metal dissolved in water. Go easy on the shampoo: it contains phthalates that could be the cause of increasing rates of genital abnormalities and testicular cancer in males. Toothpaste has cancer-causing chemicals. The risks multiply, though, when you step into the kitchen for breakfast. Fat, carbs, sugar, salt, meat, milk – all have been indicted. Are you sure you want to risk that coffee? Researchers at Brown University in the US have found that among middle-aged and older adults, light to moderate coffee drinkers had an elevated risk of heart attack in the hour after having a cup of coffee.

Coffee, a witch's brew of over 100 chemicals, has generated countless scare stories and there may be many more to come. According to biochemists Bruce Ames and Lois Swirsky Gold, 'The natural chemicals that are known rodent carcinogens in a single cup of coffee are about equal in weight to a year's worth of ingested synthetic pesticide residues that are rodent carcinogens. This is so, even though only three per cent of the natural chemicals in roasted coffee have been adequately tested for carcinogenicity.'

More than 20 years ago, the *New England Journal of Medicine* reported that 'pancreatic cancer was 2.1 times more likely among people drinking up to two cups of coffee per day; it was three times more likely among those drinking five cups of coffee of coffee a day or more . . . we estimate the proportion of pancreatic cancer that is attributable to coffee consumption to be more than 50 per cent'. Since pancreatic cancer is one of the most lethal of cancers, that warning from a reputable source must have put the wind up many coffee drinkers.

It took several years before further studies were completed, showing 'no relationship at all between coffee and the risk of pancreatic cancer or any form of cancer'. In the meantime, the health conscious were switching to decaffeinated coffee because other studies warned that regular coffee elevated cholesterol levels. It wasn't long, though, before decaf itself was condemned because industrial solvents were used to remove the caffeine. Mice dosed with these chemicals developed cancer of the stomach in larger than expected numbers.

Decaf was also claimed to raise women's risk of developing rheumatoid arthritis. Researchers followed more than 31,000 women aged 55 to 69 who were included in the Iowa Women's Health study from 1986 through to 1997. They tracked the 158 women who developed rheumatoid arthritis during that time period and compared them with women who did not develop the disease. They found that women drinking four or more cups of decaf were at more than twice the risk of developing rheumatoid arthritis. Other studies show that decaf also increases 'bad' cholesterol. Currently, well this week at least, ordinary coffee is being hailed as a wonder drink, capable of lowering the risk of type 2 diabetes and gallstones, discouraging the development of colon cancer and reducing the risk of Parkinson's disease.

So what are we to make of all this? The ups and downs of coffee health stories highlight several principles to keep in mind when trying to determine whether or not a health warning is valid. The first is that one study is never enough to establish whether or not something is bad for you. In the case of the study linking coffee and pancreatic cancer, other researchers were quick to point out that the methodology was flawed. Hospital patients were used as the control group of non-coffee drinkers, but the study ignored the fact that many had stopped drinking coffee only when they became ill – and the report made no attempt to track the pattern of coffee drinking prior to illness. In subsequent animal tests and epidemiological studies no link was found between coffee and pancreatic cancer.

Another thing to remember when assessing health scares is that mice, with the possible exception of Stuart

Little, have critical differences to human beings. Nor can the results of laboratory tests involving rodents force-fed (usually via stomach tubes) huge doses of a given substance be extrapolated to show that the tested substance causes cancer in humans. In the case of decaf, it's been estimated that human beings would have to drink approximately 24 million cups to receive the dose of the alleged carcinogenic chemicals equivalent to those fed to mice. The chemicals used to remove caffeine may indeed be carcinogenic but they are present only in microscopic quantities. It's the dose that makes the poison.

Statistics can be scary but they prove nothing. Health scares often involve epidemiology, the study of disease rates in human populations. Just because 158 women who drank decaffeinated coffee developed rheumatoid arthritis compared to women who did not drink it and did not develop the disease does not prove a connection between the two. Correlation does not prove causation. By dredging the data it may be possible to 'prove' statistically that women who wear red shoes have twice the risk of getting rheumatoid arthritis.

Scare stories almost always inflate the real risk. For example, non-smokers who are married to smokers are at a 30 per cent greater risk of getting lung cancer than non-smokers who are married to non-smokers. An increased risk of 30 per cent may sound high – but lung cancer in non-smokers is so rare that it hardly constitutes any risk at all. You may be 10 times more to contract leprosy after drinking noodle soup compared to noodle soup abstainees, but it's a risk you can afford to take. As Theodore Dalrymple points out in his book *Mass Listeria*: 'Often it is ill-appreciated that a small increase in a high risk can be more significant, from the point of view of lives lost, than a large increase in a low risk.

A one per cent increase in deaths from a disease that causes 100,000 deaths a year results in more than twice as many extra deaths as a 1000 per cent increase in deaths from a disease that causes 50 deaths a year.'

When the media are not scaring us to death, they're giving us false hope. If every 'medical breakthrough' we read about were true, we'd be so disease-free that most hospitals would by now have been converted to apartment blocks. Every week there's a story touting a 'promising' new drug, medical product or treatment. In the 1990s, for example, the hormone leptin was widely proclaimed to be the answer to weight loss. Mice injected with leptin lost 40 per cent of their body weight within a month. Soon, we were told, a leptin pill would make willpower and diet books redundant. Losing weight would be as easy as putting it on. Unfortunately, it soon became clear that leptin does not have the same slimming effect in humans that it has in mice. Xenical (orlistat), the drug that blocks fat absorption, was another false hope. Xenical seemed to promise that you could have your cake and eat it too, a sort of morning-after pill for gluttons. However, when the hype subsided, it became clear that it produced only modest weight loss. There were also unpleasant side effects, such as oily, fatty stools, the inability to control bowel movements, and gas with faecal discharge.

We are always 'on the verge of a cancer breakthrough', media reports suggest. But usually nothing much comes of it. An Australian study of cancer breakthrough reports in the *Sydney Morning Herald*, for example, identified 31 unique items over the years 1992–1994 . 'Thirteen of these 30 reports (43 per cent) were judged as not having been supported by further research in the following decade, with three (10 per cent) having been refuted, while 16 (53 per cent) were judged to remain potential breakthroughs, but more research was required. Eight breakthroughs (27 per cent) had, or would soon be, incorporated into practice.'

News stories invariably overstate the significance of what is often a single study yet to be verified by other research. Many 'breakthroughs' can be traced back to PR firms, working on behalf of biotech or drug companies intent on promoting their product or boosting their share price on the promise of preliminary research. PR agencies are incredibly helpful to busy journalists, spoon-feeding them information and lining up interviews with medical experts who are happy to simplify complex data. The fact that they or their institutions may have a financial interest in promoting the drug or treatment rarely gets a mention in the subsequent news story.

Another favourite media health story centres on raising awareness of a condition that is 'under-recognised' and 'under-treated'. For example, after decades of air travel and many millions of passengers each year taking long haul flights, deep vein thrombosis (DVT) was suddenly discovered in 2001 to be 'an under-estimated, under-diagnosed and under-treated public health threat'. By coincidence Aventis Pharmaceuticals had a new anticoagulant drug Lovenox, which could be injected prior to departure.

People who worried about DVT may also have been suffering from GAD or generalised anxiety disorder. GAD, defined as excessive and uncontrollable worry about everyday life, was a 'hidden epidemic' media reports claimed. As luck would have it, GlaxoSmithKline had just been given approval to treat GAD with its antidepressant Paxil, otherwise that would have been another thing to worry about.

Unless they are very specific and balanced, most health stories in the media can be treated as little more than speculation. 'Is someone likely to profit if I act on this information?' is a good question to ask. That's not to suggest that the media does not have a role in highlighting genuine health concerns, or that there aren't any under-estimated, under-diagnosed and under-treated public health threats. A condition that has gone largely unreported, for example, is MNS or media naivety syndrome. It's characterised by a complete failure to read between the lines.

On the Fringe

Alternative medicine
is defined as that set of
practices that cannot be
tested, refuse to be tested
or consistently fail tests.

RICHARD DAWKINS
*PROFESSOR OF THE PUBLIC UNDERSTANDING OF
SCIENCE AT OXFORD UNIVERSITY (1941–)*

THIRTY-ONE

Go Complementary, Not Alternative

Some years ago John, a 57-year-old plumber with a bad back, bad breath, constipation and chronic tiredness, consulted an iridologist. 'I went because my wife was going,' says John. 'I was pretty sceptical.' The iridologist examined his eyes with a magnifying glass and told him exactly what was wrong with him. 'I hadn't told her anything. I was so impressed. I was blown away.'

The consultation turned his life around. He followed her advice to cut his sugar intake, eat fruit, and drink lots of water. He took the herbal remedy, linseed and slippery elm, that she recommended 'to break down the hard bits in my bowel'. He was soon a new man. 'I'd been constipated all my life. I virtually educated myself reading on the toilet. I'm very happy. I'm going to the toilet beautifully now.' The bad breath has gone, and he no longer wants to sleep the afternoon away. He believes the iridologist's advice may have saved him from bowel cancer.

Iridology is one of the more absurd alternative health therapies. Iridologists claim they can diagnose any illness by looking into the iris of the eye. Iridology is based on a theory developed by Hungarian doctor Ignatz von Peczely. As a

10-year-old boy, in 1836, Peczely noticed that the iris of an owl with a broken leg had a single sharp black line in it. When the leg mended, the line disappeared. Peczely concluded that there was a causal relationship between the fracture and the iris line. When he became a doctor he found the same relationship between illness and irises in patients. Since the 1970s, when the theory made a comeback, iridology has gown in popularity.

John agrees that the basis of iridology is 'very strange. But she got it right.' The question, though, is how? When John is questioned more closely about the consultation, other factors emerge. While waiting for the consultation, he felt hungry and ate four chocolate fish. That chocolate smell would have been detectable while she examined his eyes. A possible diagnosis: high sugar intake. John admits to yawning frequently during the consultation (high sugar intake is linked to chronic tiredness). The bad breath might indicate constipation. John says he had suffered from a bad back for most of his life, a condition that may have been evident from his posture. There is also the scattergun effect relied on by psychics and 'mind readers'. Mention 10 possible diagnoses and selective thinking leads us to remember only the 'hits' and dismiss all the apparent misses. In fact, what makes some iridologists successful is that they are able, consciously or unconsciously, to 'read' the patient and have good clinical skills. An American study demonstrated this. When shown photographs of 143 irises without ever meeting the patients, the iridologists did no better than chance in making a diagnosis.

For John, however, the fact that iridology may be pseudoscience does not matter. 'All I can say is it worked for me. I must be a healthier person now than I was.' The experience has left him more open to alternative health therapies. John doesn't go to the doctor very often. 'But I went the other day. I had a list of five things. He says, "Oh, we haven't time for all that." Doctors treat symptoms. He takes your blood pressure, examines your physique, and thinks, "Here's a healthy man, get him out of here, I've got sick people to see." Whereas this woman seemed to look inside me and see that I was in need of attention.'

John is just one of millions who are becoming increasingly alienated by conventional medicine and are seeking out alternative therapies. Most doctors don't have the time to investigate the root causes of a patient's complaints and settle for treating the symptoms. There are also many chronic conditions that conventional medicine is not good at treating, such as neck and back pain and rheumatoid arthritis. Some vague conditions such as chronic fatigue syndrome, fibromyalgia and irritable bowel syndrome may be psychosomatic and more likely to respond to treatment by a sympathetic alternative healer than a sceptical or frustrated doctor.

As Professor Raymond Tallis points out in *Hippocratic Oaths*, his sturdy defence of conventional medicine, it may take time for an illness to become distinct enough to be able to diagnose it correctly. But sick people want answers right away. 'The disempowerment of illness is sometimes blamed on the institutions – and above all on the individuals who work within them – who, because they are not instantly available and cannot provide instant answers, keep one waiting in ignorance. The knot of waiting, impotence and uncertainty at the heart of sickness contributes to many patients' discontent with medicine.'

Conventional medicine may not work for everyone,

but alternative medicine may be even less effective. Some alternative treatments may appear to work because of the placebo effect (a factor in conventional medicine as well, of course). Many illnesses are self-limiting: they will go away without any treatment. If your earache disappears after your feet have been massaged by a reflexologist, you will be encouraged to believe that the two events are connected.

Conditions such as arthritis, allergies and multiple sclerosis come and go. People who usually seek help in the down cycle often credit the remission to the treatment when it is simply part of the natural cycle of the disease. It's what is known as the *post hoc ergo propter hoc* (after this therefore because of this) fallacy, a piece of faulty logic that has led many of us astray. The temptation is to believe that if A occurs before B, A is the cause of B. A boss, for example, may assume that because his employees laugh at his jokes they must be funny. It ain't necessarily so. Diseases, such as cancer, can also go into spontaneous remission; one oncologist reported that it occurred in 12 out of 6000 cases he treated. Such events can fool both healer and patient into believing the treatment worked.

It's often assumed that alternative treatment is risk-free because it's usually based on a natural substance or process. But there's nothing particularly benign about nature. The stones and pips of apricots, plums, cherries, peaches, apples and pears all contain glycosides, which if eaten release potentially lethal doses of cyanide. Some herbal remedies have similar toxic effects to prescription drugs. If something has the power to do you good, it also has the potential to do you harm. Alternative treatment needs to be subject to the same risk–benefit analysis as conventional medicine, argues Professor Edzard Ernst, Britain's first Professor of Complementary Medicine. Ernst is also a co-author of *The*

Desktop Guide to Complementary and Alternative Medicine: An Evidence-Based Approach, one of the most authoritative books on the subject. Though a strong advocate of complementary medicine's role in healing, he is not blind to the harm it can cause.

Acupuncture has caused deaths and serious complications through infection and trauma, and chiropractic manipulation can be risky. One US study found it was the number one reason for people suffering stroke under the age of forty-five. While therapies such as acupressure, reflexology, homeopathy and spiritual healing may cause no direct harm, they can have an indirect risk if they lead people to delay seeking proven treatment for a life-threatening condition. 'We recently encountered a non-medically qualified CM practitioner who noticed a pigmented lesion on her arm and self-medicated with homeopathic remedies without consulting her doctor, even though the lesion increased in size. When she finally went to see her physician, an advance malignant melanoma was diagnosed: tragically, she died shortly afterwards,' wrote Ernst in the journal, *Diabetes Care.*

The evidence for many alterative treatments is often non-existent or doesn't stack up. You have to rely on testimonials, which are subjective and notoriously unreliable. However, as Ernst says, 'Many complementary therapies have been "field tested" for hundreds of years on millions of people. The resulting evidence amounts to a kind of plausibility that science neglects at its peril.' But just because it's old does not make it valid. Witchcraft was practised in many cultures for millennia but that does not mean it's not superstitious mumbo-jumbo.

One of the tests of any valid system is surely that it changes and evolves. As we learn more, some things are discarded and new ones take their place. In all disciplines the obsolescence of knowledge is a measure of progress and no more so than in medicine. You'd be aghast if your doctor suggested bloodletting as a treatment for your high blood pressure instead of using hypertension drugs. Yet many people are happy to submit to alternative treatments that haven't changed for hundreds of years. As John Diamond noted in his book, *Snake Oil*, 'The alternativists complain – against the evidence – about orthodoxy's hidebound unwillingness to change, while at the same time taking a perverse pride in the antiquity of their own techniques. I've never come across an herbalist who has revealed that a remedy used by his professional forebears has been discovered, after all, not to work or a homeopath complaining that his craft is still stuck in the rut ploughed by homeopathy's founder two hundred years ago.'

When alternative treatments do work their effectiveness may often be more due to the diagnostic skills and intuition of the practitioner rather than to the validity of the practice. The risk is that some alternative healers don't know their limitations or have such a warped view of conventional medicine that they put patients' health at risk by steering them away from proven treatment such as chemotherapy. Hippocrates' dictum should be the watchword of all healers, conventional and alternative: 'First do no harm.'

THIRTY-TWO

Resist the Lure of the Health Store

It's easy to be seduced by the charms of health-store medicines. Who could resist Throat Myst: 'For this exceptional blend we started in the damp chilly hills of Scotland where the elderberry herb comes highly recommended. Then we added slippery elm, marshmallow root, licorice, propolis, echinacea, golden seal and vitamin C'? Surely a healing drop, and more natural and pleasant to take than nasty chemicals like benzocaine.

Natural, though, doesn't always mean safe or sensible to use. Otherwise health stores would be doing a roaring trade with all-natural products like heroin – 'This ancient calmative derived from the beautiful poppy plant, organically grown on the Himalayan foothills and harvested by local tribesmen and their families in the time-honoured way', as the blurb might put it. Nor does natural mean chemical-free. We owe our existence to the life-sustaining chemical soup that makes up the Earth and its atmosphere. Pick up an apple, for example, and you are ingesting more than 200 chemicals from its aroma alone. Claims that 'all natural' is always healthier should be taken with a pinch of sodium chloride.

It's undeniably reassuring, though, when you can

pronounce the name of the medicine you're taking. One of the pleasures of browsing in a health store is savouring the names: Devil's Claw, Horehound Root, Mandrake, Lady's Slipper, Blue Cohosh, Horsetail, Blessed Thistle. The health store is the place to discover all the ailments you never knew you had, and get in touch with your inner organs. Do I need a dose of cranberry that 'stops harmful bacteria attaching to the bladder lining'? The detoxifying 'Authentic Sheep Sorrel' on discount is tempting, but then so too is the Prostaguard because, as it says, 'A well-fed prostate . . . is a happy prostate!' The BV (bee venom) Skin Cream might do wonders for my arthritis but wouldn't it be more natural, not to mention a lot cheaper, just to aggravate a few bees in the garden? I would be more reassured about the efficacy of the 'Insomnia Formula' if it didn't say on the bottle 'won't cause drowsiness'.

Though their advertising hype does sometimes stretch credibility, it would be wrong to dismiss all herbal remedies as snake oil. St John's Wort has been used for more than 2000 years to treat mental disorders and other conditions. Legend has it that the plant (or wort in old English) grew from the blood that fell from St John's beheading. Taking a medication with a legend attached to it is guaranteed to make you feel better. In clinical studies St John's Wort has been shown to be as effective as antidepressants like Prozac for mild to moderate depression with fewer side effects. (Which isn't saying a lot since studies show that antidepressants are little better than placebos.) It's also said to be good for procrasti-nation, though researchers haven't got around to verifying that yet.

Frankincense, the aromatic resin from the Boswellia tree used to make incense, was one of the gifts of the Magi, but is also useful to treat arthritis and joint injuries. Boswellia has been shown to be more effective than a placebo in treating osteoarthritis of the knee.

Feverfew has shown promise as a treatment for migraine headaches though further studies are needed to confirm the initial findings. Feverfew is claimed to be effective against fever and colds if it's gathered with the left hand as the name of the patient is spoken aloud and without a glance behind. This too needs further study.

The Mayans made a tonic from the berries of the saw palmetto plant, and now there is evidence that it is just as effective as the medication finasteride in treating enlarged prostate. It may also prevent male pattern baldness. Horse chestnut for varicose veins, ginger for morning sickness, ginkgo for dementia, folate to prevent birth defects, aloe vera for constipation – dozens of natural remedies have proven to be effective medicines or are showing promise.

Herbal remedies, however, are classed as dietary supplements rather than medicines in many countries and are not subject to the same regulations that control pharmaceuticals. That means it can be difficult to be sure how much active ingredient is in a pill as this can vary from brand to brand and even from batch to batch. An analysis of six different capsules and four liquid extracts of St John's Wort, for example, found a huge variation in potency. Herbal remedies also sometimes include impurities or unlisted ingredients. Some Chinese medicines have been found to contain pharmaceuticals such as chlorpheniramine (an antihistamine) and sildenafil (Viagra).

On the whole, though, herbal remedies are safe to use. A 2003 editorial in the *British Medical Journal* put it in perspective: 'Even though herbal medicines are not devoid of risk, they could still be safer than synthetic drugs. Between

1968 and 1997, the World Health Organization's monitoring centre collected 8985 reports of adverse events associated with herbal medicines from 55 countries. Although this number may seem impressively high, it amounts to only a tiny fraction of adverse events associated with conventional drugs held in the same database.'

It's unknown, though, how many adverse events go unreported, as studies show many people are reluctant to reveal to their doctors that they use herbal remedies. That's a worry because the biggest danger in self-medicating with herbal medicines is the interaction with conventional drugs. Fewerfew, garlic and ginger can lead to excessive thinning of the blood in people who take warfarin. Kava, a herb used to treat anxiety, can cause gastrointestinal and liver problems, and is dangerous when used with sedatives, sleeping pills, alcohol, antipsychotics and drugs to treat Parkinson's disease. St John's Wort can cause you to burn faster in the sun, especially when combined with other photosensitisers such as tetracyclines, and can interact with the heart medication digoxin and with oral contraceptives. Gingko biloba, used to increase circulation and memory, is dangerous if taken with aspirin or warfarin and may cause spontaneous and/ or excessive bleeding. Echinacea will increase the risk of liver toxicity when taken with arthritis drugs. Flaxseed can affect the potency of some heart drugs by rendering them un-absorbable. Ginseng should not be used when you're taking drugs to control high blood pressure. And so on. Not all herbal medicine and conventional drug interactions have been documented.

Don't expect much guidance from health-store staff either. Most have no formal training in nutrition or health care. Many investigations over the years have shown advice from health-store staff to be unsafe or inappropriate. For example, one woman who had a stomach complaint was advised to take peppermint oil, good for some stomach problems but very bad for the hiatus hernia that she actually had. In a 2003 study of 34 Canadian health stores, researchers trained to act as customers whose mothers were suffering from breast cancer, asked staff for product recommendations. None of the 33 different products recommended was supported by evidence of effectiveness. Sixty-eight per cent of the health store staff did not ask whether the patient was taking prescribed medication and only 8.8 per cent discussed the adverse effects of the products. Less than a quarter pointed out that the products might interact with prescribed drugs.

Both health stores and supermarkets turn over a tidy profit from the sales of vitamins. Until recently it's always been assumed that taking vitamins was safe in recommended doses. The conventional wisdom was while they were unnecessary for anyone eating a balanced diet, they were unlikely to cause harm since in most cases any vitamin excess was excreted in urine. However, a 2007 Danish study has found that even modest doses of the common antioxidant vitamins beta carotene, vitamin A, vitamin C (ascorbic acid), vitamin E and selenium either singly or in combinations could increase the risk of mortality in some people. Since we know so little about the risks versus benefits of taking herbal remedies and vitamin supplements, we'd be better to spend our money on high quality fresh food.

Regular visits to the health store can take your hypo-chondria to the next level. Instead of bog standard worries like cholesterol and high blood pressure, you'll soon be able to fret over imbalances in gut flora, weakened digestive juices, sluggish liver function, nutrient deficiencies, intestinal overgrowth of *Candida albicans*, inadequate levels of neuro-transmitters, early red blood cell destruction, levels of inositol in your spinal fluid, and reduced cerebral circulation. You may find yourself lying awake at night wondering if your membranes are becoming leaky predisposing you to food intolerance or whether you're losing too much calcium, magnesium and phosphorus through urination. Have you tried Easy Sleep, a non-addictive herbal combination of valerian, passion flower, scullcap, hops and wild lettuce?

THIRTY-THREE

Avoid Cures 'They' Don't Want
You to Know About!

Millions die of cancer each year yet there are all-natural cancer cures on the Internet that work for between 95–98 per cent of sufferers. What is it about Googling 'cancer cure' that people don't understand? Well, maybe most people realise that if you have a cure for cancer you don't have to write in caps and pepper your prose with exclamation marks.

When we're sick or desperate, though, our critical faculties may atrophy. Only that may explain why, for example, author Kevin Trudeau sold five million copies of his book, *Natural Cures 'They' Don't Want You to Know About*. Hucksters like Trudeau, a convicted fraudster, perpetuate the myth that there is a vast conspiracy preventing us from accessing natural cures for cancer and other life-threatening diseases. In a sequel, *More Natural Cures Revealed*, he writes: 'I have heard with my own ears how Big Pharma, the food industry, and the oil industry are working together with governments and media outlets around the world. I have been in over sixty countries, yet there are no stamps of evidence in any of my passports. I have been to Area 51 in Nevada. (The existence of this top-secret military installation is still denied by the US government.) This is where much of our technology has been developed. Area 51 houses most extraterrestrial artefacts, including a working spacecraft and dead alien bodies. I've seen these things with my own two eyes.'

Claiming a conspiracy exists is a favourite ploy of those who peddle snake oil because it deflects attention away from the real issues of whether or not their products work. While it may be true that Big Pharma will use all its clout and even resort to dirty tricks to protect its multi-billion-dollar industry and to disparage natural products, it does not follow that there's a cabal of pharmaceutical companies and doctors actively suppressing natural cures.

Maybe it's the growing acceptance of alternative and complementary therapies or the pervading influence of the Internet, but quackery is flourishing as well as it did in its heyday, the 19th century. Promising bigger breasts and penises is a sure-fire way to extract money from the gullible. In 2003, an Arizona company was shut down and its owners jailed for selling breast enlargement pills that guaranteed an increase of 'two or three cup sizes' in weeks, and penis enlarger pills called Longitude, which 'will make your penis grow until you are satisfied with your new size' (with commendable consideration for its customers, the company suggested discontinuation of the pills when the penis extended to nine inches in length to avoid discomfort to partners). Other enhancing pills in the product range included Stature (to increase height by up to four inches) and Long Jack (a golf game improver). The company had sales of $74 million over two years.

One reason people fall for these scams is that they are under the impression that health products are better regulated than they are and the government would not allow them on the market if they didn't work. In fact, companies can get away with a lot if they are clever enough not to be too explicit in their claims about their products' efficacy.

It's not just pills and herbal remedies that rake in the cash. Quack medical devices have been regular big sellers. The Super-Zapper Deluxe, a device developed by naturopath Dr Hulda Clark, sells for $189. It was claimed to be effective in killing bacteria, viruses and parasites in the human body and to be effective against chronic infections, cancer, and AIDS until the US courts prohibited Clark from making unsubstantiated claims.

Pricing is always a challenge for quacks. Pitch your price too low and people won't take you seriously; pitch it too high and the punters will be reluctant to give it a try. The ACU-STOP 2000!, for example, a rubber device to align the pressure points in your ears believed to control appetite, cost only 17 cents to make and sold for $39.95, which is probably the least you could charge to have any credibility in the marketplace. Unfortunately the makers were unable to substantiate their claims that the device could decrease or suppress appetite and it had to be taken off the market. (A better bet, perhaps, if you want to lose weight effortlessly is 'sanitized tape worms', a popular slimming product of the 1930s, which promised, 'Eat! Eat! Eat! And Always Stay Thin! No Diet, No Exercise!')

It's their desire to help people find the easy way out by harnessing new technology that often gets these medical entrepreneurs into trouble. In their enthusiasm they oversell the product. For years doctors and Olympic athletes have been using electronic muscle stimulation (EMS), a process that uses a low electrical current to stimulate the muscles to contract and relax. When a muscle contracts as a result of electronic stimulation, the chemical changes that take place within the muscle are very similar to those that occur during normal exercises. In other words all you have to do is throw a switch to get your muscles moving. It wasn't long before someone came up with the idea of strapping an EMS machine to your tummy to work on your abs while watching TV, or as the ad put it, 'a gym of bulky expensive exercise equipment' shrunk into 'a little electronic miracle the size of a pack of matches'. Alas, the little miracle didn't live up to its claims that '10 minutes with Fast-Abs is equivalent to doing 600 sit-ups'. While it did create muscle contractions, they weren't deep enough to develop the 'awesome abs' promised by the maker.

There's nothing like an electric current, though, for what ails you. Until it was taken off the market in the US, The Stimulator was just the thing for pocket or purse. Essentially an electric gas barbecue drill igniter fitted with finger grips, it gave a small electric shock when applied to the skin. If you believed in it enough, it could cure your headache, back pain, arthritis, stress, earache and other ailments. For the complete electrical experience, though, you need to take 'the Kremlin Pill', a Russian-invented capsule that emits electric pulses inside you and stimulates the internal organs. At $50 each, it's fortunate that the pill is reusable. However, 'the less pleasant part of the experience is retrieving the capsule so that it can be cleaned, sterilized and swallowed again. Rubber gloves and a sieve are recommended for the retrieval process.'

The invention of electricity generation in the 19th century led to an explosion of dubious medical devices. One enterprising quack came up with the idea of electric spectacles that sent a small current to the optic nerve, so that 'the organ of sight was restored to its original strength'. Electropathy became extremely popular, and was touted as a cure for every ailment including mental illness. Many of these weird and wonderful machines are now in Bob McCoy's Museum of Questionable Medical Devices in Minnesota.

With worldwide access to the gullible through the Internet, quackery will continue to thrive – and entertain. My favourite is the 'Eternal Life Rings and Eternal Foot Braces' invented by Alex Chiu. The devices, consisting of 'rare or ceramic magnets', are worn during sleep and guarantee that you will live forever. You get your money back if not satisfied. You can't get fairer than that.

THIRTY-FOUR

Try the Panacea in the Pantry

When drug companies have good news, their PR agencies go into overdrive bombarding the media with information and mounting publicity campaigns on TV and in the press. But when an everyday food like vinegar proves to have healing properties, there's a lot less media coverage.

In 2005, Carol Johnston, a Professor of Nutrition at Arizona State University, discovered that taking two tablespoons of vinegar in water before a meal works just as well as taking diabetes medication. Five studies in the 1980s showed that vinegar might be useful in controlling diabetes, but Johnston was the first to show that it works. Type 2 diabetics and those with pre-diabetes need to control their blood sugar levels because their bodies cannot utilise insulin effectively to move sugar from blood into cells. Over time, high levels of glucose in the blood can lead to heart disease, kidney disease, blindness and other complications. In her study, Johnston found that vinegar cut the blood–glucose concentrations of diabetics in the first hour after a meal by 25 per cent. People with pre-diabetic symptoms who took vinegar before a meal had lower blood glucose than even healthy volunteers who also drank vinegar.

The same effect can be achieved with anti-diabetes drugs, but in addition to the expense, they can also have side effects, such as gastrointestinal disturbances. Johnston also discovered a significant bonus in people taking vinegar: weight loss. Over the four-week trial, volunteers taking vinegar before two meals each day lost on average 0.91 kg (2 lb).

The snag, of course, is that vinegar is hardly anyone's idea of an aperitif. It's possible to enjoy vinegar in pickled foods or in a salad, but the solution may lie in vinegar capsules containing sufficient acetic acid, which Johnston believes is the anti-diabetic ingredient in the vinegar. Scientists are now developing an encapsulated form of vinegar that they hope will be just as effective as ordinary vinegar.

The medicinal properties of vinegar have been known long before Jack was a boy and his mother bound his head in vinegar and brown paper. The folk remedy is still popular for swelling and painful heel spurs. Vinegar heads believe that there's very little that vinegar is not good for, from spraying on your underarms as a deodorant to gargling for a sore throat, to relieving the pain of sunburn and to preventing infection from new body piercing. In developing countries vinegar is used as a way to detect cervical cancer. The cheap and effective screening method involves washing the cervix with vinegar, viewing it with a flashlight and freezing any white spots (possible cancer cells) with carbon dioxide.

The usefulness of vinegar seems endless. Want to select the right multivitamin? To be effective, multivitamin tablets need to disintegrate and dissolve completely. If after dropping a multivitamin into half a cup of vinegar and stirring occasionally it has not disintegrated after 20 minutes, it's time to try another brand. (Vinegar, of course, is not only an aid to health, but an all-purpose cleaner of windows and greasy bench tops, a stain remover and weed-killer.)

Garlic is the other Swiss Army knife of healing. Legend has it that when Tutankhamun's tomb was opened six perfectly preserved garlic bulbs were found among the other priceless treasures. It's not known what King Tut intended to use the garlic for in the afterlife – but it has no end of uses in this one. Garlic is reputed to be a cold and flu preventative, although how much of its effectiveness is due to its medicinal properties and how much to the fact that it keeps other people at a distance is not clear.

Hanging a string of garlic bulbs around your neck might act as a warning to the odd vampire or troll, but it won't do much for your health. To get benefit from garlic you have to slice or crush it. At that moment it releases an enzyme called allinase that converts the molecule alliin into allicin. You can tell this is happening because that's when garlic begins to smell like garlic. Garlic has been described as the 'ultimate cardiovascular herb' because it thins the blood, lowers blood pressure and lowers cholesterol. It may also have a role in cancer prevention. Epidemiological studies have found that in areas of the world where people eat a lot of garlic (and onions) there is a decreased incidence of cancer.

But the benefits of garlic don't end there. During World War I it was used to treat wounds. Recent research suggests that garlic blocks the action of certain enzymes that help infectious microbes survive in host tissue. Because of its antibiotic properties one natural therapist recommends threading a peeled garlic clove and inserting it in your ear if you have earache. ('What's that? Will you speak up, I've got a garlic clove in my ear!')

Garlic has been tried in all orifices. A peeled (but unbruised) clove of garlic inserted in the rectum after a bowel movement will apparently do wonders for haemorrhoids by disinfecting the area and bringing down the swelling. By the time you get through a bulb or two you could be haemorrhoid-free.

In ancient Greece, garlic was used to determine fertility. A peeled clove of garlic was placed in a woman's vagina and left overnight. If she had the smell of garlic on her breath the next morning it was considered that she was able to conceive a child. A large clove of garlic has been a popular folk remedy for treating vaginal infections such as thrush. Garlic is said to stimulate sexual desire, which is why some religious orders of monks and nuns eliminated it from their diet. It's claimed that certain chemicals in garlic cause mild irritation in the urogenital tract, which has a very pleasurable and stimulating effect.

Garlic has many more mundane uses. It's reported to be effective against athlete's foot and sunburn, will stimulate hair growth, cure cold-sores, help clear up coughs, do wonders for sinus, relieve sore throats and jock itch, prevent insect bites, control outbreaks of oral and genital herpes, can be useful in weight control and help with hangovers. It can also be used to relieve constipation in your horse, will prevent mites on your budgie, act as an effective flea repellent and cure worms if you add it to your cat or dog's diet.

If vinegar is hard to swallow, the drawback with garlic is, of course, the smell. Garlic is so powerful that it can enter your system by being absorbed through the skin. So, even if you're massaging your feet with garlic oil to ease your blisters, you will still have garlic breath. The traditional way to get rid of garlic breath is to chew parsley. If you don't want to spend the next hour picking out little green bits from your teeth, try chewing a coffee bean, a mint leaf or a cinnamon stick. Enteric-coated garlic tablets leave no odour because the garlic is absorbed in the small intestine, but it's not clear how effective garlic supplements are.

Ginger is another spice that is showing promise as a healing agent. It's already known to ease nausea and is being investigated as treatment to lessen the effects of chemotherapy. Recently, powdered root ginger has been shown to be as effective as chemotherapy in stopping the growth of ovarian cancer cells in laboratory tests, but it's too early to say whether eating more ginger would offer any protection against cancer.

Another condiment commonly found in the pantry may also have health benefits. Curcumin, a compound found in turmeric, could, research suggests, slow down neurodegenerative diseases such as Alzheimer's disease. In India where turmeric is most widely used in cooking, Alzheimer's affects just 1 per cent of people over the age of 65 living in some villages. Researchers also found that curcumin, which is an antioxidant and anti-inflammatory, had other health benefits: it aids digestion, helps fight infection and guards against heart attacks.

When traditional remedies like vinegar, garlic and turmeric are validated by science, it's tempting to believe that all time-honoured natural healing methods must have something to them. Why else would they have survived? Well, for one thing, the placebo effect, the observation that belief in a treatment enhances its effectiveness, ensures that any treatment in any age was guaranteed to work for some people. There is also good money to be made resurrecting ancient remedies and selling them to a gullible public.

Though about a quarter of all medicines used today have plant origins, there are many herbal remedies that are complete duds or, worse, dangerous to take. Just because something is natural does not mean it's safe. Herbs such as comfrey and chaparral that used to be very popular are no longer much used because they have been shown to cause liver damage. Those in the natural health industry dismiss such warnings as an attempt to discredit natural products, pointing out – quite rightly – that the risk associated with pharmaceuticals is many times greater. However, pharmaceuticals at least are required to undergo some clinical testing; natural products at present are not because they are deemed to be dietary supplements. Without testing and standardised manufacturing, it's hard to know if dietary supplements contain contaminants or what their potency is.

Consumers in the middle are left to make up their own minds. It's worth adopting the motto of the editors of the *Journal of the American Medical Association*: 'In God we trust. All others must have data.' One useful source of independent information is *Tyler's Honest Herbal: A Sensible Guide to the Use of Herbs and Related Remedies*. Varro E. Tyler was, until his death in 2001, a recognised world authority on plant drugs (herbs) and their uses. Tyler was scathing about the use of words like 'natural' and 'organic' to ratchet up the price on medicines, which are in essence chemical compounds. 'The word "natural" applied to such materials identifies only a source and does not imply a degree of superiority or inferiority,' he noted. He acknowledged that while many herbs such as echinacea and ginseng have been shown to have definite therapeutic value, many others are potentially toxic. There is danger, too, in self-diagnosis and self-medication to say nothing of the hazard to the patient's pocketbook, he pointed out. 'For all of these reasons, you are less likely to receive value for money spent in the field of herbal medicine than in almost any other.'

THIRTY-FIVE

Increase Your Pulling Power

Feeling out of sorts? You could put it down to 'Magnetic Field Deficiency Syndrome'. Headaches, back and neck pains, insomnia, heaviness of head and general lassitude are just some of the symptoms of this syndrome, according to Japanese magnet therapist Dr Kyochi Nakagawa. It's known that the Earth's magnetic field has decreased by about 6 per cent since 1830 and evidence suggests that it may have lost 30 per cent of its pull over the past millennium. If this sounds like your particular deficiency, you could try a magnetic mattress; 10 million Japanese sleep on them every night.

Magnet therapy has also become more popular in the West. Britain's National Health Service is now subsidising the use of a magnetic leg wrap to heal ulcers after a double-blind randomised trial showed it helped patients to heal faster. A double-blind study at Baylor College of Medicine in Houston, Texas, found that magnets reduced pain in post-polio patients, and more studies to determine if magnets can relieve pain are being funded by the US Office of Alternative Medicine. Natural Standards, a respected body that sifts the evidence for complementary and alternative therapies, states that pulsed electromagnetic fields can improve the healing of fractures in the bones of the lower leg, electromagnetic stimulation therapy can be useful for patients with urinary incontinence, and magnetic shoe insoles are a promising treatment for numbness and diabetic foot pain.

It may be some time before your doctor suggests novel uses for your fridge magnets, but magnet therapy is already a billion-dollar industry. Cherie Blair, Bill Clinton and Sir Anthony Hopkins are reported to be satisfied customers. Many golfers and professional athletes swear by their magnet therapy devices. However, physicist James D. Livingston, author of *Driving Force: The Natural Magic of Magnets*, has argued that aside from the placebo effect there may be other explanations why magnetic therapy devices seem to work. A magnetic back brace, for example, may provide mechanical support through localised warming 'and through constant reminder to the ageing athletes that they are no longer young and should not overexert their muscles'. A British study that examined the use of magnetic pulsing to stimulate bone growth found that the same results could be obtained when the device was switched off and concluded that it was the enforced inactivity, not the pulsed magnetic field, that was responsible for improvement.

The popularity of a treatment does not always mean that it's effective. Magnet therapy was wildly fashionable in the 18th century. Viennese physician Franz Anton Mesmer became a sensation all over Europe because of the many cures he achieved with the use of magnets. Mesmer later decided it was 'animal magnetism', a magnetic force within his own body that was flowing between him and his patients and curing them. In 1784 a French Royal Commission investigated his claims of animal magnetism and concluded that it was no more than the power of suggestion. However, as Livingston has pointed out, Mesmer's mysterious animal magnetism later evolved into other forms of therapy including hypnotherapy, chiropractic, therapeutic touch and Christian Science healing.

With the development of technology, such as electricity in the 19th century, magnet therapy enjoyed a resurgence in popularity. Dr C. J. Thacher, president of the Chicago Magnetic Company, was a leading exponent of magnet therapy, claiming it 'will cure every curable disease no matter what the cause'. The company sold a large range of magnetic garments or you could buy the complete set containing over 700 magnets, which would 'furnish full and complete protection of all the vital organs of the body'. Thacher, like many magnet therapists who came after him, claimed that magnetism affected the iron in the blood. However, the iron in blood is very different from, say, the iron in a frying pan. Iron in the blood is magnetic but the iron atoms are isolated within the red blood cells and would not be affected by magnets.

Magnet therapists also argue that it's important to have the right magnets and have them facing in the right direction. North (negative) poles are said to relieve pain and reduce swelling, whereas south (positive) poles accelerate growth indiscriminately, promote anxiety and make sleep less restful. Unipolar magnets have flat surfaces and expose the subject to just one field; bipolar magnets expose the skin to both fields simultaneously. Both types of magnets have their proponents. However, the magnets in most therapy products are too weak to penetrate more than a few millimetres in the body so are unlikely to have much effect.

Nevertheless, our bodies function through electrochemical processes and create a very weak magnetic field. As Livingston says, 'We are all electromagnets.' It's not known how or if a lot of the electromagnetic fields we encounter every day have an effect on the body. A 1997 study found that low-level electromagnetic fields, equivalent to those found in people's homes, could reduce the effect of the cancer drug tamoxifen, at least in test-tubes. Tamoxifen is a synthetic hormone used to prevent the recurrence of breast cancer. In his book, *Cross Currents*, Robert O. Becker, an authority on bioelectromagnetics, warned against many common household appliances, including electric blankets, electric clocks and television sets. The bigger the TV screen, the stronger the electromagnetic radiation. Rats exposed to four hours of TV a day showed retarded growth, changes in brain function, and in males the size of the testicles was significantly reduced. (And that's on top of the atrophy of the critical faculties caused by the actual programmes.)

Electromagnetic pollution is increasing at an alarming rate. Computers, mobile phones, iPods, PDAs; even our cars produce electromagnetic fields from dozens of sources, from power-steering to mirror motors. There's no evidence that these do us any harm. But even as sceptical a scientist as Livingston is not convinced the magnetic fields in today's environment are totally harmless. He writes: 'In 1982 two researchers who failed to find any effects of strong magnetic fields on humans concluded their study with puzzlement: "Magnetism is certainly a remarkable force, and we find it very difficult to understand why it seems to have no influence whatever on the human body and its wonderfully delicate neuroelectric mechanism." I agree. It seems likely that magnetic fields much stronger than the earth's magnetic field could affect our biological processes, sometimes in a helpful manner, sometimes harmful.'

Like most living things, though, the human body is

diamagnetic, weakly repelled by magnetic fields. However, a powerful magnet will still have an effect. In 1996, scientists used a high-field electromagnet to levitate a frog. It's technically possible to build a magnet big enough to levitate human beings, but you would ruin all their credit cards in the process.

Magnetic fields have long been thought to have a powerful – and useful – effect on the brain. Cleopatra, legend has it, wore a lodestone on her forehead to combat ageing. Tibetan Buddhists place magnets on the skulls of novice monks to improve their concentration and learning ability. Transcranial magnetic stimulation (TMS) is now used to treat a variety of illnesses such as schizophrenia, depression, Parkinson's disease and obsessive compulsive disorder. TMS works by creating a magnetic field that passes through the brain, affecting neurons in a particular area. It's no use, though, filling your beanie with fridge magnets; a TMS device consists of special magnetic coils that must deliver its charge within a thousandth of a second to a specific area of the brain. TMS was originally used to test for nerve damage. Like a small hammer, it can check your reflexes. Directed to the motor cortex just under the scalp, the magnetic field can make your thumb twitch, or your leg jerk.

Australian researchers led by neurologist Allan Synder have been using TMS to temporarily shut down parts of the brain, in effect, creating a small lesion. This has the remarkable effect of enhancing artistic and mathematical abilities in volunteers in much the same way – but not to the same extent – that certain skills are amplified in brain-damaged savants. By using a magnetic field to temporarily impair the part of the brain that enables us to think conceptually, we are able to see things in a raw unprocessed state. 'Remember that old saw which says that we only use a small part of our brain? Well, it might just be true. Except that now we can prove it physically and experimentally,' Synder told the *New York Times*.

One of the most useful applications of magnets has been to find our way around the world. The Chinese invented the compass around the year 300 BC. However, birds, bees and other animals have magnetic sensors in their bodies to enable them to use the Earth's magnetic field for navigation. In the 1970s, scientist William Keeton put this to the test by gluing small magnets onto the backs of homing pigeons, Sure enough, the birds became disoriented and lost their way. Zoologist R. Robin Baker was convinced that humans' sense of direction is also derived from the Earth's magnetic field. To test his theory he devised Keeton-like experiments involving students at Manchester University. The students were blindfolded and driven in a roundabout fashion about 48 km (30 miles) from Manchester. They were then asked to point in which direction their dorms were located. Students with magnets on their heads did less well in the test than students with similar non-magnetic objects on their heads. The lesson is clear: if you're given to wearing a fridge magnet on your head to relieve headaches, it's a good idea to take it off before you go out. Otherwise you may never find your way home.

THIRTY-SIX

Take the Piss

I've never been a big fan of urine. At boarding school we had to queue up to empty our chamber pots each morning, a routine I've since observed only in old prison movies. As a parent, the early years were measured out in soggy nappies rank with ammonia. Like most people I've always associated urine with faeces, waste products that are best disposed of quickly before they breed disease.

In fact, for thousands of years and in many cultures urine has been prized as a remedy for all sorts of ailments. In recent years it has been making a comeback. There have been several world conferences on urine therapy. New books on the subject have been published, some of which are appearing on public library shelves. The most famous modern advocate of urine therapy was Indian Prime Minister Morarji Desai, who drank a cup of urine each day and lived a healthy life until the age of ninety-nine.

'Morarji cola', as it's sometimes dubbed, isn't to everyone's taste, but there's really nothing to justify the revulsion most people feel at the thought of swallowing it. Being a waste product does not mean that a substance is toxic or harmful: it just means that the body cannot absorb it at the present time. Urine is actually 95 per cent pure water and five per cent solids, mostly urea and salt. The urine from a healthy animal or human is sterile. Nor does it have any odour until the urea is broken down by organisms in the environment, giving off that characteristic ammonia smell.

The Chinese used urine as a medicine for more than 2000 years, and Hindu Ayurvedic medicine, which dates back to 1000 BC also makes wide use of urine. The Aztecs used it to wash wounds, and some American Indians used urine for regular skin care. In Europe, seventeenth- and eighteenth-century doctors prescribed urine for gout and the 'vapours', the hysterical giddiness common among women in those times. In Elizabethan times the English and Dutch would toast each other's health with urine mixed with wine. Urine drinkers are fond of pointing out that the amniotic fluid that surrounds human infants in the womb is primarily urine – so we all began life as urine drinkers. Christian fundamentalists should feel a duty to practise it as the *Bible* says so: 'Drink water from your own cistern, flowing water from your own well' (Book of Proverbs, 5:15).

We spend billions on drugs while our own natural panacea is flushed down the toilet, advocates argue. There is said to be little urine can't cure or alleviate: AIDS, allergies, snake bites, asthma, heart disease, eczema, fatigue, jet lag, baldness, hangover, depression, insomnia ... the list goes on – and on. Pierre Fauchard, the eighteenth-century founder of dental science, was a believer in mouthwashes. One should rinse one's mouth each morning, he advised, with several spoons of one's own freshly voided urine to ensure good healthy teeth.

Though the cure-all claims are the stuff of pure quackery, there is some substance in the claim that urine contains healing agents. Urea is an antibacterial and antifungal agent and has been used to treat human infection since the 1930s. It is also a major component of moisturisers and creams for cracked skin. During the Korean War, soldiers peed in their helmets and soaked their feet in urine to heal and toughen the skin. Its antiseptic effect apparently helped clear up ruptured blisters.

Alchemists once tried to extract gold from urine because they thought that's what gave it its distinctive yellow colour. However, it took modern pharmaceutical companies to find a way of making money out of it. Urine is a good source of hormones: the urine of postmenopausal Italian nuns has been used to manufacture Pergonal, a drug used to stimulate ovulation in women and sperm production in men. Urokinase, a urine ingredient, is used in drug form as a blood-clot dissolver for unblocking coronary arteries. You would need to drink a lot of urine to benefit, though. In the US, urokinase is produced by collecting and filtering urine from Porta-John portable toilets. The 14 million gallons of urine collected produces 2 kg (4.5 lb) of urokinase, enough to unclog 260,000 arteries.

So does it make sense to drink urine? Some argue that it is biologically illogical to take into the body what has already been excreted as waste. However, in his book *The Water of Life* J. W. Armstrong draws an analogy with composting: 'Rotting dead leaves, when dug back into the soil, provide valuable mineral salts to nourish new plant life. The same principle holds good for the human body.'

The consensus is that the best urine to drink is a fresh, midstream draught first thing in the morning. As an experiment I swallowed half a glass and it was not nearly as revolting as I'd imagined – a warm, odourless, slightly salty tipple. Like Guinness, though, it's obviously an acquired taste. I remember feeling better that day. Was it a placebo effect or the fact that morning urine contains high levels of melatonin, the wonder hormone that aids sleep, alleviates jet lag and has proven tranquillising effects? Recent research suggests melatonin can reduce abdominal pain, bloating and other symptoms of irritable bowel syndrome (IBS).

In Siberia, the Koryak people drank the urine of people who had eaten fly agaric mushrooms to communicate with spirits. There's apparently a lot of mileage in hallucinogenic mushrooms: potency does not decrease until the seventh drinker because the kidneys secrete the psychedelic compound unaltered. Gym junkies, perhaps, could save themselves a fortune by finding a weightlifter prepared to share their steroid-enriched body fluid. In general, though, it's advisable to stick with your own urine, and it's not a good idea to imbibe if you're already on prescription medicines.

For most people urine will probably remain the medicine of last resort, though it does seem a pity not to make use of such rich waste. Urine is more than 50 per cent nitrogen and is said to be as potent as chemical fertiliser. Some gardeners use diluted urine on pot plants and flower beds. If you're going to pee on your garden make sure it's on well-mulched or well-aerated soil or on piles of leaves. And well away from the neighbours.

THIRTY-SEVEN

Have a Cuppa

The trouble with pleasures that have been proved to be medicinal is that they stop being medicinal all too quickly. Chocolate contains powerful antioxidants but 28 gm (1 oz) three times a week is all that's recommended. Red wine is good for your heart – but only if you stop after the second glass. However, there's one healthy pleasure that remains unrestricted – tea drinking. Tea has long been touted as a health drink. One old Chinese proverb says: 'Drinking a daily cup of tea/ Will surely starve the apothec'ry.' The notion of tea as a health drink lingers on in the names of popular British brands. Typhoo is Chinese for doctor, and PG Tips is short for pre-gestive tips. 99 Tea was also known as Doctor's because 99 was the number on old prescription forms. Now there's a growing body of scientific research to support many of the health claims made for tea.

Tea can take its place with fruit and vegetables as generators of antioxidant activity. Like fruit and vegetables, tea contains polyphenols, particularly in the form of flavonoids. Polyphenols are believed to reduce the risk of heart disease. Flavonoids are said to slow down atherosclerosis. One cup of tea contains about 200 mg of flavonoids. Drinking three cups of tea a day over two weeks increases the concentration of flavonoids in the blood by 25 per cent. Tea also contains catechins, which have been used to treat hypertension by inhibiting the action of an enzyme that constricts blood vessels. Tea may also decrease the blood's tendency to form clots, which can lead to strokes and heart attacks.

There is also some evidence that tea can help protect against cancer. Preliminary research by the National Centre for Toxicological Research in the US demonstrated that theaflavins and polyphenols extracted from tea inhibited the growth of human pancreatic and prostrate tumour cells. Another study published in the *International Journal of Cancer* indicated that men who drink between two and three cups of tea a day may reduce the risk of developing prostate cancer by up to 30 per cent compared with non-tea-drinkers. Studies in Japan and China have linked tea drinking with lower incidences of stomach and liver cancer. In Sweden, researchers looked at the eating and drinking habits of 61,057 women aged between 40 and 76 over a three-year period and found that drinking at least two cups of tea a day reduced the risk of ovarian cancer by nearly 50 per cent.

L-theanine, an amino acid found in tea plants and particularly in green tea, is said to have calming effects and to modify the stimulating effects of caffeine and enhance alertness. An article published in the journal *Psychopharmacology* found that tea drinking lowers levels of cortisol, the hormone that floods our system when we are stressed, causing our blood pressure to rise and heart to race. Catechins in green and black tea have been shown in the laboratory to destroy amyloid, the protein believed to cause Alzheimer's disease, though human clinical studies are yet to be done. According to one British study, women aged between

65 and 75 who drank at least one cup of tea a day had higher bone density in spine and thighs, areas that are susceptible to fractures caused by osteoporosis. A US study of 35,000 showed that women who drank at least two cups of black tea a day were 40 per cent less likely to develop urinary tract cancer and 68 per cent less likely to develop cancer of the digestive tract than women who were not tea drinkers.

One lesser-known health benefit of drinking tea is its effect on oral health. A cup of tea contains between 0.3 and 0.5 mg of fluoride. Beverages, mainly tea, account for 85 per cent of our fluoride consumption. Making tea with fluoridated water doubles your fluoride intake if you drink four or five cups a day. About 34 per cent of the fluoride we get from tea is retained in the oral cavity, helping prevent tooth decay. Other components of tea – tannins, flavonoids, catechin, caffeine and tocopherol – also have protective effects, inhibiting the growth of bacteria and increasing the acid resistance of tooth enamel. Tea may also protect against oral cancer. One study found that heavy smokers who drank five cups of green tea a day for four weeks had fewer damaged cells in their mouths.

Tea may offer protection against food poisoning and diseases such as dysentery. Some researchers believe that it acts as a mild germicide in the digestive tract. In laboratory tests, powdered tea added to eight kinds of bacterial cultures (including *Salmonella* and *Staphylococcus*) prevented them from developing colonies of bacteria. A cuppa may be just what you need to get over the effects of being zapped by radiation. Russian researchers say that tea helps the body excrete harmful radioactive strontium 90 before it settles in the bones. The Chinese claim that tea will help absorb strontium 90 even after it has lodged in the bones. Good news if you live within missile range of North Korea. According to the Chinese, tea may also contribute to longevity. Chinese researchers have found that jasmine and oolong tea more than doubled the life of fruit flies, the human equivalent of 150 years. And we are closer to the fruit fly than many of us would like to think, sharing 60 per cent of genes.

And don't just drink tea. Put it in your socks (to prevent athlete's foot), on your eyes (to relieve tiredness), on cuts (if there is nothing more medicinal to wash with), on sunburn, on insect bites (to relieve discomfort), and on tired feet. The one thing not to do with tea is to use it to wash down pills. Some of the 400 chemical compounds identified in tea may cause an adverse reaction when combined with certain drugs.

It may not be true that all teas have the same beneficial effects. Though black teas and green teas come from the same *Camellia sinensis* plant, the leaves are fermented to different degrees. Though both contain powerful antioxidants, green tea is often cited as the more effective in helping prevent cancers. Tea brewed from loose leaves and left to steep for about five minutes has more antioxidant power, and iced tea can be just as healthful. Herbal teas may have other benefits, but they don't contain the health-promoting polyphenols contained in green, black or red teas.

The real excitement in health-conscious tea drinkers, however, centres on rooibos, or red bush tea. Rooibos grows only around the village of Clanwilliam in South Africa. Rooibos is naturally caffeine-free, and according to one study its antioxidant properties are up to 50 times more potent than those in green tea. There's not a lot rooibos won't do for your health. It relieves insomnia, nervous tension, mild depression, stomach cramps (including colic), constipation, and allergic symptoms such as those caused by hay fever. It's good for eczema, nappy rash and acne when applied to the affected area, and may even help you recoup after a hangover.

Since tea is the most popular beverage in the world, though, you have to ask, why are we all not a lot healthier? Well, maybe we don't drink enough of it or maybe the many health claims based on inconclusive or preliminary research have been overstated by the tea industry. The Irish, for example, are the world's greatest tea drinkers, consuming on average six cups a day, yet Ireland ranks only 21st in life expectancy among the world's nations. Tea may indeed help prevent certain cancers but the effect may be quite small. It's also possible that as a recent study suggests, the health benefits of tea drinking are negated when we add milk because the caseins in milk reduce the concentration of catechins. Regardless of how we take it though, it still has benefits. It increases our fluid intake, and if we take it with milk, keeps up our calcium levels. And it's no exaggeration to say that tea has saved millions of lives simply because making it requires boiling water, which prevents countless diseases. Let's have a cuppa.

Finally ...

Be careful about reading
health books. You may
die of a misprint.

MARK TWAIN
US WRITER AND HUMORIST (1835–1910)

THIRTY-EIGHT

Think Before You Swallow

The paradox is that the more time and thought we devote to staying healthy, the less likely we are to be so. That's because we may be more likely to take prescription medication or self-medicate, and we may be putting ourselves at risk for very little benefit. We're also more likely to be swayed by the marketing of health products of dubious value, more likely to try the next fad diet, and more likely to be made more anxious and fearful by the latest media health scare or disease awareness campaign.

This book has been about trying to avoid those traps and focusing instead on making life more pleasurable and satisfying. For the generation now enjoying life in their eighties, health was a normal state, not something you had to constantly work at. Gym workouts were for athletes or narcissists. Food was something to savour or fill your stomach, not a medicine to prevent heart disease or cancer.

While cutting back on meat, eating more vegetables and jogging for an hour a day may make you less susceptible to certain diseases, it may not do you much good if you don't enjoy it and are constantly beating yourself up for failure to live up to the 'healthy' ideal. Though we're always reminded to eat healthily, no one can say with any certainty whether it's going to help us avoid disease or live longer. As writer Michael Pollan has pointed out, nutrition is enormously complicated: 'Even the simplest food is a hopelessly complex thing to study, a virtual wilderness of chemical compounds, many of which exist in complex and dynamic relation to one another, and all of which are in a constant state of changing from one state to another.' Is cooking destroying the nutrients we need or are the foods we eat at the same time preventing their absorption? 'Drink coffee with your steak, and your body won't be able to fully absorb the iron in the meat,' writes Pollan. Is it the lack of a specific nutrient in Western diets that makes us susceptible to cancers or the wrong ratio of Omega 6s to Omega 3s? A low-fat diet, we were constantly told, would protect against heart disease and breast cancer, but in 2006 a US Women's Health Initiative study of nearly 50,000 women over eight years found no links.

Today's dogma is tomorrow's heresy. And that's as it should be, because real science is continuously evolving, discarding current theories and testing new ones, unlike the pseudoscience of alternative medicine, which remains static and unchanging. But constant change does highlight the absurdity of altering our eating habits to conform to the latest nutritional advice. Remember the oatbran craze of the 1980s? Now it's probiotics. It's your gut bacteria that's making you sick, stupid.

Apart from smoking-related illness, we can't say with any certainty what causes most diseases or why some people get them and others don't. Nevertheless, a healthy lifestyle has become elevated to the level of a religion. If we smoke or eat junk food or laze on the couch we are not merely being dumb; we are bad people. 'In this secular age focusing upon one's diet and other lifestyle choices has become an alternative to prayer and righteous living in providing a means of making sense of life and death,' writes Deborah Lupton in her book, *The Moral Imperative of Health.* ' "Healthiness" has replaced "Godliness" as a yardstick of accomplishment and proper living.' The US, as usual, has been at the forefront of this trend with faith-based diet books. *What Would Jesus Eat? The Ultimate Program for Eating Well, Feeling Great, and Living Longer* by Don Colbert includes Jesus' favourite desserts (low calorie rather than sinfully fattening, no doubt).

Everybody, of course, should be free to practise their own religion even if it has no higher ideal than body maintenance and the pursuit of longevity. It's when devotees attempt to foist their faith on others or discriminate against unbelievers that it becomes problematical. In the UK, for example, primary-care health trusts in East Suffolk are denying patients knee and hip replacements if they have a Body Mass Index (BMI) of over 30. And in a survey of British doctors conducted by the British Medical Association almost 40 per cent of doctors said that obese patients, smokers and heavy drinkers should be excluded from treatments. Australian Associate Professor Matthew Parris has argued that denying smokers joint replacement surgery, breast reconstructions and some other types of elective surgery is justified because the operations are more risky and costly when performed on smokers (unlikely to be true in all cases). As baby boomers age, there will be more calls for rationing of health resources and those who don't conform to current health doctrines will be sent to the back of the queue.

Children are not exempt from the healthy lifestyle crusade. Some Australian preschools and kindergartens are searching children's lunches for contraband such as chocolate frogs, lollies, cakes and fruit roll-ups. In the UK, fat children are likely to find themselves on the child protection register alongside victims thought to be at risk of sexual or physical abuse. In extreme cases fat children have been placed in foster care. It's hardly surprising that eating disorders are becoming more common, even in children. In developed countries, some estimates suggest 1 in every 200 young women has anorexia nervosa and up to 3 in every 100 have bulimia nervosa. A New Zealand study found that 52 per cent of females are dissatisfied with their body, 37 per cent of girls have dieted (from as young as seven years old) and 14 per cent of boys have dieted.

Healthy living is a choice, not a virtue. It does not make you a better person, nor should it be considered a marker for good citizenship. As historian Robert N. Proctor points out in his book *The Nazi War on Cancer*, there have been few more health-conscious, socially responsible and environmentally aware governments in recent times than the Third Reich. Hitler, like Franco and Mussolini, was a non-smoker and took a personal interest in anti-smoking campaigns. Smoking was banned in many public places and tobacco advertising was strictly controlled. Smoking was branded 'lung masturbation', and smokers who regularly took time off work because of 'cigarette stomach' (gastritis or ulcers) could be remanded to a nicotine-withdrawal clinic.

The Nazis launched massive campaigns to encourage the early detection of cancers. Women were instructed in how to examine their breasts for cancer, and men were advised to check their colons as often as they would check the engines of their cars. Nazi politicians talked about 'health as a duty' (not so dissimilar from the nineties' catchcry about 'taking responsibility for your own health'). The Nazis were also strong advocates of wholegrain bread (bakeries were required by law to produce it), raw fruit and vegetables, and less meat. Soya beans became politically correct, earning the nickname 'Nazi beans'. 'Nutrition is not a private matter!' warned a Hitler Youth manual. Hitler himself was a vegetarian, who described meat broth as 'corpse tea', favoured pure olive oil, and worried that the increasing consumption of whale oils was diminishing the population of whales. Himmler was somewhat similar: he was strongly opposed to 'refined flour, sugar and white bread'. The wholemeal biscuit, though, was favoured by Rudolf Hess, who took along his own 'biodynamic' vegetarian food when invited to dinner, a habit that apparently got up Der Führer's nose.

This is not to denigrate or dismiss healthy living or public health campaigns by association – the Nazis, for example, were commendably decades ahead of their time in promoting workplace health and safety, at least for Aryans – but to underline the fact that a healthy society is not necessarily one that places great importance on bodily health but one that cherishes the freedom of its citizens. It's worth observing that it was Winston Churchill, the obese Olympic-class smoker and drinker – a bottle of wine for breakfast was not exceptional – who lived to 90 and made a greater contribution to the world than the abstemious health-obsessed Adolf Hitler. As psychologist and author Peter Marsh has said, 'We need some bad habits in order to retain our subscription to the human race.'

That's not to argue that *What Would Churchill Drink? The Ultimate Program for Getting Pissed, Feeling Great, and Living Longer* should be our guide to health. As I've tried to show in this book, there is a middle ground between the irrational rejection of the benefits of modern medicine and the obsessive concern for health that threatens to blight our lives. It's the middle path that most of us instinctively choose but can no longer pursue with confidence because of the incessant voices urging us to exercise more, eat more vegetables but less fat, stay out of the sun, lose weight, drink less, and scrutinise our body for moles and lumps.

It's wise, though, to be alert to changes in our bodies and take prompt action if concerned. There's no better health advice than that on the side of every packet of aspirin: 'If symptoms persist, see a doctor'. However, it doesn't follow that screening for disease is necessarily a good thing. Like any other medical intervention there are both benefits and risks. For example, The Cochrane Collaboration, one of the most reliable sources of healthcare information, carried out a major review of breast-cancer screening in October 2006. The review examined seven trials involving a total of half a million women. 'The review found that mammography screening for breast cancer likely reduces breast cancer mortality, but the magnitude of the effect is uncertain, and screening will also result in some women getting a cancer diagnosis even though their cancer would not have led to death or sickness ... for every 2000 women invited for screening throughout 10 years, one will have her life prolonged. In addition, 10 healthy women, who would not have been diagnosed if there had not been screening, will be diagnosed as breast cancer patients and will be treated unnecessarily. It is thus not clear whether screening does more good than harm.'

H. Gilbert Welch, a US Professor of Medicine and author of *Should I Be Tested for Cancer?*, questions whether early disease detection is a good thing. 'To understand this, you need to understand that each of us harbours early forms of disease,' he wrote in the *Washington Post*. 'Even in middle age, many of us who feel well have evidence of diabetes, heart disease, osteoporosis, hepatitis, vascular disease and cancer. Just because we harbour these early forms of disease doesn't mean that they will ever affect our health. Some diseases progress so slowly that people die of other causes long before the diseases generate symptoms. Other diseases may not progress at all. Unless we were tested, we'd never have known we were sick.'

Prostate cancer is a classic example, he says. Around half of all men at age 60 will have microscopic evidence of prostate cancer yet only 4 in 1000 will die of it within 10 years. While screening would save some lives it would turn many more men with non-progressive disease into cancer patients.

In *The Tyranny of Health*, British GP Michael Fitzpatrick writes 'that there is a high degree of scepticism about the value of such health interventions among the medical profession. However, recognising the strength of the health promotion consensus, solidly backed by government funding, medical vested interests and compliant journalists they think it best to keep their reservations to themselves ... a spirit of "not in front of the children" governs debate as medical science is subordinated to political expediency.' In other words we're being lied to. As Professor David Seedhouse, Director of New Zealand's National Centre for Health and Social Ethics, has said in his book *Health Promotion: 'Philosophy, Prejudice and Practice'*, health promotions often contain half-truths, exaggerations and opinion masquerading as fact. 'But it is apparently all right for health promoters to deceive.' It's for a good cause, after all.

Whether you are being lied to for commercial gain or in the interests of public health, the result may be the same, putting your health and wellbeing at risk. Make your own decisions based on the best evidence you can find. It's your body. It's your life.

Think before you swallow.

Further Reading

1 NEVER SUPERSIZE YOUR WARDROBE

Dale Atrens, *The Power of Pleasure – Why Indulgence is Good For You and Other Palatable Truths*, Duffy and Snellgrove, 2000

Paul Campos, *The Obesity Myth: Why America's Obsession with Weight Is Hazardous to Your Health*, Gotham Books, 2004

David Knight and Steven Bratman, *Health Food Junkies: The Rise of Orthorexia Nervosa – The Health Food Eating Disorder*, Broadway Books, 2004

2 KEEP YOUR NOSE CLEAN

Susan F. Rudy, *Nuances of Nasal and Sinus Self-help*, Trafford Publishing, 2004

Michael Stoddart, *The Scented Ape: The Biology and Culture of Human Odour*, Cambridge University Press, 1990

3 TALK TO THE HAND

John T. Manning, *Digit Ratio: A Pointer to Fertility, Behavior and Health*, Rutgers University Press, 2002

John Napier, *Hands*, Princeton University Press, 1993

5 KEEP IN TOUCH

Diane Ackerman, *A Natural History of the Senses*, Random House, 1995

Ashley Montagu, *Touching: Human Significance of the Skin*, Harper & Row, 1987

7 JUST WALK

Rebecca Solnit, *Wanderlust: A History of Walking*, Verso Books, 2006

8 SLEEP ON IT

Deirdre Barrett, *The Committee of Sleep: How Artists, Scientists, and Athletes Use Dreams for Creative Problem-Solving – And How You Can Too*, Crown Publishers, 2001

Paul Martin, *Counting Sheep: The Science and Pleasures of Sleep and Dreams*, Flamingo, 2003

9 TAKE YOUR OWN SWEET TIME

Peter Axt and Michaela Axt-Gadermann, *The Joy of Laziness: How to Slow Down and Live Longer*, Bloomsbury, 2005

Edward M. Hallowell, *CrazyBusy: Overstretched, Overbooked, and about to Snap! Strategies for Coping in a World Gone ADD*, Ballantine Books, 2006

Carl Honoré, *In Praise of Slow: How a Worldwide Movement Is Challenging the Cult of Speed*, Orion, 2005

10 CHOOSE TO BE HAPPY

Mihaly Csikszentmihalyi, *Flow: The Classic Work on How to Achieve Happiness*, Rider, 2002

Wayne Froggatt, *Choose to Be Happy*, HarperCollins New Zealand, 2004

Jonathan Haidt, *The Happiness Hypothesis: Putting Ancient Wisdom to the Test of Modern Science*, Basic Books, 2005

Martin Seligman, *Authentic Happiness: Using the New Positive Psychology to Realise Your Potential for Lasting Fulfilment*, Nicholas Brealey, 2003

11 GIVE AWAY YOUR TIME

Robert D. Putnam, *Bowling Alone: The Collapse and Revival of American Community*, Simon & Schuster, 2001

13 TAKE A SONIC TONIC

Don Campbell, *The Mozart Effect: Tapping the Power of Music to Heal the Body, Strengthen the Mind and Unlock the Creative Spirit*, Hodder & Stoughton, 2002

14 GET DOWN TO EARTH

Donald Norfolk, *The Therapeutic Garden*, Bantam, 2001

15 READ FOR YOUR LIFE

Wendy Kaminer, *I'm Dysfunctional, You're Dysfunctional: The Recovery Movement and Other Self-Help Fashions*, Perseus Books, 1992

Jack J. Leedy, *Poetry Therapy*, Lippincott, 1968

Steve Salerno, *SHAM: How the Gurus of the Self-Help Movement Make Us Helpless*, Nicholas Brealey, 2006

16 SCREEN YOUR GENES

Carol Krause, *How Healthy Is Your Family Tree? A Complete Guide to Tracing Your Family's Medical and Behavioral Tree*, Prentice Hall, 1994

17 SURVIVE THE FAMILY

John R. Gillis, *A World of Their Own Making: Myth, Ritual and the Quest for Family Values*, Harvard University Press, 1997

Oliver James, *They F*** You Up: How to Survive Family Life*, Bloomsbury, 2003

20 TAKE YOUR GLASSES TO THE SUPERMARKET

Walter Gratzer, *Terrors of the Table: The Curious History of Nutrition*, Oxford University Press, 2006

Michael Pollan, *The Omnivore's Dilemma: The Search for the Perfect Meal in a Fast-Food World*, Bloomsbury, 2006

21 WORK TO LIVE

Madeleine Bunting, *Willing Slaves: How the Overwork Culture Is Ruling Our Lives*, Harper Perennial, 2005

Joanne B. Ciulla, *The Working Life: The Promise and Betrayal of Modern Work*, Times Books, 2000

22 TUNE INTO THE WEATHER

Manfred Kaiser, *How the Weather Affects Your Health*, Michelle Anderson, 2002

23 DON'T BE IN IT FOR THE LONG HAUL

Diana Fairechild, *Jet Smarter: The Air Traveler's RX*, Flyana.com, 1999

24 TRY NOT TO TAKE GLOBETROTTING LITERALLY

Philip M. Tierno, *The Secret Life of Germs*, James Bennett, 2004

Jane Wilson-Howarth, *Bugs, Bites and Bowels*, Cadogan Guides, 2006

26 LEARN THE DIFFERENCE BETWEEN A PILL AND AN iPOD

Ray Moynihan and Alan Cassels, *Selling Sickness: How Drug Companies Are Turning Us All into Patients*, Allen & Unwin, 2005

Darian Leader and David Corfield, *Why Do People Get Ill?*, Hamish Hamilton, 2007

27 OVERCOME YOUR CHOLESTEROLPHOBIA

Uffe Ravnskov, *The Cholesterol Myths: Exposing the Fallacy That Cholesterol and Saturated Fat Cause Heart Disease*, New Trends Publishing, 2001

28 KEEP TAKING THE RIGHT TABLETS

Marcia Angell, *The Truth About the Drug Companies: How They Deceive Us and What to Do About It*, Random House, 2005

30 READ BETWEEN THE LINES

Theodore Dalrymple, *Mass Listeria*, Andre Deutsch, 1998

Richard A. Deyo and Donald L. Patrick, *Hope or Hype: The Obsession with Medical Advances and the High Cost of False Promises*, AMACOM, 2005

Stanley A. Feldman and Vincent Marks, *Panic Nation: Unpicking the Myths We're Told About Food and Health*, John Blake, 2006

31 GO COMPLEMENTARY, NOT ALTERNATIVE

Rob Buckman and Karl Sabbagh, *Magic or Medicine? An Investigation of Healing & Healers*, Pan Books, 1995

John Diamond, *Snake Oil and Other Preoccupations*, Vintage, 2001

Raymond Tallis, *Hippocratic Oaths: Medicine and Its Discontents*, Atlantic Books, 2005

34 TRY THE PANACEA IN THE PANTRY

S. Foster and V. E. Tyler, *Tyler's Honest Herbal: A Sensible Guide to the Use of Herbs and Related Remedies*, Haworth Press, 1999

35 INCREASE YOUR PULLING POWER

Robert O. Becker, *Cross Currents: Perils of Electropollution, the Promise of Electromedicine*, Jeremy P. Tarcher, 1991

James D. Livingston, *Driving Force: The Natural Magic of Magnets*, Harvard University Press, 1997

36 TAKE THE PISS

J. W. Armstrong, *The Water of Life: A Treatise on Urine Therapy*, Vermilion, 2005

Carol Seinfeld, *Liquid Gold: The Lore and Logic of Using Urine to Grow Plants*, Green Books, 2004

FINALLY ...

Michael Fitzpatrick, *The Tyranny of Health: Doctors and the Regulation of Lifestyle*, Routledge, 2000

James Le Fanu, *The Rise and Fall of Modern Medicine*, Abacus, 2000

Robert N. Proctor, *The Nazi War on Cancer*, Princeton University Press, 2000

David Seedhouse, *Health Promotion: 'Philosophy, Prejudice and Practice'*, John Wiley, 2000

Index

Index

Index